Y0-BBC-731

EMBRACEABLE YOU

A Guide for Orthodontic Patients
and Their Parents

JAY WEISS, D.M.D.

Health Sciences Publishing Corp.
New York
1975

Library of Congress Cataloging in Publication Data

Weiss, Jay, 1927-
  Embraceable you; a guide for orthodontic patients and their parents.
  Includes bibliographical references.
  1. Orthodontia. 2. Teeth—Abnormities and deformities. I. Title.
  [DNLM: 1. Orthodontics—Popular works. WU400 W431e 1974]
  RK521.W4   617.6'43   72-4351
  ISBN 0-88238-603-4

Library of Congress Catalog Card No. 72-4351

Copyright © 1975 by Health Sciences Publishing Corp.

Printed in the United States of America by
Meilen Press Inc., New York, N. Y.

For Bill Tutin:
Who loved books and for Gene and
Joan who loved Bill

ACKNOWLEDGMENTS

The assistance and counsel of friends and colleagues who read all or part of the manuscript is gratefully acknowledged. These included Mr. Merwin Fuchs, Dr. Milton Glatzer, Mrs. Lillian Kutscher, Dr. Irwin Mandel, Mrs. Anne McCarthy, Dr. Merrill Stern, and Mrs. Lillian Weiss. My office assistants, Mrs. Cecilia Kohl, Miss Elida Ponce, and Mrs. C. Raymond submitted to an additional amount of torment, sometimes without complaint, during the time this book was being written. In addition, Mrs. Kohl labored patiently typing the manuscript.

Finally, it was my good fortune to work with Roberta Halporn, a real professional. To all, my warm thanks.

Despite this generous guidance, mistakes of omission and commission doubtless persist. For them I accept *both* blame and responsibility.

TABLE OF CONTENTS

	PAGE
Introduction	ix
Everything You've Always Wanted to Ask	xi

Chapter One:
    From Ancient Egypt to Health Insurance 1

Chapter Two:
    Malocclusion, What Is It? 7

Chapter Three:
    The Emotional Importance of Teeth 11

Chapter Four:
    Workers in the Field: Who Treats Malocclusion? 19

Chapter Five:
    The Diagnostic Decision 1: Gathering Information 25

Chapter Six:
    The Diagnostic Decision 2: To Extract or Not to Extract? 31

Chapter Seven:
    Further Diagnostic Adventures 39

Chapter Eight:
    Final Diagnostic Adventures—The Doctor's Dilemma 47

	PAGE
Chapter Nine:	
Dental Data	55
Chapter Ten:	
The "Right" Age to See an Orthodontist	67
Chapter Eleven:	
Molar Mechanics	73
Chapter Twelve:	
But Sometimes Those Gadgets Don't Work at All	87
Chapter Thirteen:	
Now You See Them, Now You Don't	99
Chapter Fourteen:	
The Role of Surgery in Orthodontics	109
Chapter Fifteen:	
Calculated Risks and Risky Calculations	121
Glossary	137
References and Notes	151

Illustrations ....*precedes page 67*

INTRODUCTION

> "now . . . the public challenges the traditional paternalism of medicine in which the doctor's word and deed go unquestioned."
>
> L. K. Altman, *New York Times,* December 5, 1972.

The stirrings of change that Bob Dylan heard "blowing in the wind," that Charles Reich saw "greening America," and that other writers like Philip Slater hoped would enrich our lonely existence will surely lead to modifications in the practice of medicine and dentistry in this country. Some adjustments have already begun. But the pace is probably going to accelerate. A movement that insists patients have a right to control the destiny of their own bodies has grown out of the struggle for civil and human rights that has been gathering force since the close of World War II. Most people will no longer meekly submit to authoritative pronouncements from any source no matter how well intentioned, superbly trained, or thoroughly anointed with ancient status. There is no reason why they should. This humanistic revolution as reflected in medicine and dentistry will liberalize give and take between doctor and patient. In the past, lanes of communication between the two players in the health game have too often been one-way, with the doctor telling and the patient listening. The street should be transformed into a highway, and traffic should be encouraged to flow in both directions.

In order for any patient or parent to exchange views intelligently with a physician or dentist, he must be supplied with basic information. Clarifying issues won't change the fundamental roles of doctor as dispenser and patient as receiver, but it may help both parties to understand what is expected of them. This book offers some data for one specialized field of dentistry, orthodontics, whose importance is likely to grow in our post-industrial society.

Such an increased awareness is desirable because the issues confronted in the orthodontic encounter transcend questions of dental health. Not only do orthodontists and their patients deal with crooked teeth, they are also concerned with basic human values. How a person looks can have a great deal to do with how he feels about himself, how much he thinks he is worth. The orthodontic process can be responsible for enormous changes in the face the patient presents to the world.

In *The Informed Heart,* Bruno Bettelheim has commented that ". . . barring an individual from a part in decision-making on matters that deeply concern him tends to create a feeling of impotence which we call being subject to tyranny."[1] If the pages that follow can provide information which will contribute to the selection of *informed* choices in orthodontics they will have played a modest part in dispelling that feeling of impotence and repelling that burden of tyranny.

EVERYTHING YOU'VE ALWAYS WANTED TO ASK ... WELL, ALMOST EVERYTHING

> What is the answer? [I was silent.]
> In that case, what is the question?
>
> Gertrude Stein, Last words, from
> Alice B. Toklas, *What is remembered.*

Confronted with some dazzling new feature of 20th century life, like a computer or space travel, Americans readily concede the value of the thing but aren't always exactly sure what it's all about. Orthodontics is one of those vaguely mysterious subjects that touch the lives of many middle class citizens who learn much of the vocabulary without fully understanding it. Precisely what does a dentist mean, for instance, when he hints darkly that you have a bad bite? (For an answer, see Chapter 2.) Some other frequently encountered questions are listed below with references to pages where answers can be found. Alice, Gertrude, are you listening?

1) How can teeth be moved? Aren't they attached to the jaw bones? (See Chapter 9.)

2) How long does orthodontic treatment take? (See Chapter 11.)

3) Will it hurt? (See Chapters 11 and 12.)

4) How much will it cost? (See Chapters 5 and 11.)

5) Can braces hurt your teeth in any way? (See Chapter 15.)

6) What are the chances of teeth moving back again after the appliances have been removed? (See Chapter 15.)

7) What's the retainer for? How long is it worn? Do you need *two* retainers? One for each jaw? (See Chapter 11.)

8) At what age should treatment start? (See Chapter 10.)

9) Can adults be treated? (See Chapter 11.)

10) Won't teeth straighten by themselves as the child grows? (See Chapter 6.)

11) What should be done about thumb sucking? (See Chapter 7.)

12) Are any other habits important to the alignment of teeth? (See Chapter 8.)

13) Should we depend on our regular dentist to decide when to go to an orthodontist or can we arrange the check up ourselves? (See Chapter 4.)

14) Will braces make the teeth hard to clean and cause cavities? (See Chapter 15.)

15) Why do braces have to show? (See Chapters 11 and 13.)

16) Why must wires be changed? Why must patients go so often for visits? (See Chapter 11.)

17) Why are there different types of braces? (See Chapter 11.)

18) Won't third molars cause teeth to get crooked again? (See Chapter 9.)

19) What are rubber bands for? (See Chapter 11.) How about the night braces? (See Chapter 11.)

20) Why do some patients have to have teeth removed? (See Chapter 4.)

21) Will braces interfere with talking? (See Chapter 12.)

Everything You've Always Wanted to Ask xiii

22) Will they interfere with eating? (See Chapter 12.)

23) How much parental guidance is needed during the treatment period? (See Chapter 12.)

24) Why can't family dentists straighten teeth? Is it really necessary to go to a specialist? (See Chapter 4.)

25) What should be done about a baby tooth that is lost prematurely? (See Chapter 10.)

26) Will I have to eat any special kinds of food or restrict my diet when I am wearing braces? (See Chapter 12.)

Chapter One

FROM ANCIENT EGYPT TO HEALTH INSURANCE, A SHORT HISTORY OF ORTHODONTICS

> Picasso had just painted a picture of a naked dental hygienist in the middle of the Gobi Desert . . . And then the war came and Hemingway went to Africa to do a book . . . Gertrude Stein moved in with Alice Toklas and I went to New York to see my orthodontist . . .
>
> Woody Allen
Second Woody Allen record.

"Looks don't mean a thing," Ring Lardner once commented bitingly, "only about ninety per-cent." Judging from the homage paid to movie stars and assorted beauty and home-coming queens or the steadily rising stocks of the cosmetics industry, Americans in general tend to agree with him. Their interest in appearance may account for the spiraling success of the specialized field of dentistry called orthodontics. Like Helena Rubinstein and the Avon lady, the orthodontic supply houses have gone public. Seemingly unaffected by the erratic ups and downs of the economy, business has been steadily good for the dentists who straighten the teeth of the nation's children.

What's it all about? Orthodontists are dental specialists whose job is to cure malocclusion, the defect which is variously described as buck-teeth, under-shot jaw, bad bite, fangs, or snaggle teeth. While its wide popularity is recent, the craft is itself by no means a modern invention, like heart transplants. In one way or another the Romans, the Incas, and the Egyptians may all have tried their hands at the rudimentary dental art. The procedure has, fortunately, lost much of its painful sting since the time of

Joseph Fox, Surgeon Dentist Extraordinary to Their Royal Highnesses, the Dukes of Kent and Sussex, who observed in 1814, that, "Extraction of the teeth is required . . . to prevent or remedy irregularity in the arrangement of the permanent teeth . . ." He warned that speed was of the gravest importance. In cases where a child needs to have more than one tooth removed, ". . . there is great difficulty, after the extraction of one . . . to persuade it to submit to a second operation." [1] Therefore, the alert surgeon would be careful to remove the second tooth before his patient realized what had happened to the first one.

Orthodontists no longer have to do their work so swiftly, like thieves in the night. Indeed, a principal complaint leveled against them is that it takes so long to complete treatment, usually about two years, give or take several months. The other chief complaint, of course, is that they charge so much. As far as the quality of their efforts goes, however, the general public has lately been reasonably satisfied. In this age of increasing technical competence, orthodontists, like other craftsmen, are growing more and more proficient. It wasn't always thus.

Only fifty years ago Calvin Case, one of the American fathers of orthodontics, lamented that "the practice of orthodontia was beginning to be feared by many of our best orthodontists as more or less a failure." [2] Although practitioners were learning how to get teeth straight in those days, they didn't know how to keep them that way. Fortunately, new stabilizing techniques have since been introduced. Such early fumbling is understandable since the science of orthodontics had just gotten started, a few years before, right here, in the United States. In the fertile soil of a nation that nurtured a brilliant band of tinkerers like Henry Ford and the Wright brothers, orthodontics, a highly mechanical enterprise, haltingly emerged. Inventive geniuses like Case and Edward Hartley Angle, building on the pioneering efforts of Norman Kingsley and John Farrar, proclaimed system after system, one more intricate than the other. All of these innovators were as American as baseball and their infant art remains to this day a curiously American undertaking. Nowhere else in the world are orthodontic services so much in demand, so well executed, and so richly rewarded. As far as the equity of the availability and the distribution of orthodontic care, there is considerable room for debate since this commodity, like many other health services is largely reserved for those who can pay for it. But with the advent of union and other health insurance plans and the imminent arrival of some governmental health scheme it is falling within the reach of increasing numbers of people. As Hixon and Klein put it in a journal article, "The last 50 years have seen orthodontic service move across the socio-economic class spectrum from a luxury item into almost all segments of society." [3]

As far as the earlier, pre-American know-how days, one British writer blithely observes that "It has been known for at least two thousand years that teeth could be moved from one position in the mouth to another by the application of prolonged force." [4] The hard evidence for any actual use of this principle before relatively modern times is scanty. One Phoenician lady, discovered in a tomb in Sidon, had delicate wires encircling several teeth. They may have been put there to correct an irregularity, but the more likely possibility is that they served to hold false teeth in place, in itself an impressive accomplishment for a dentist who dismissed his last patient 600 years before Christ was born. Bronze dental instruments, some of them quite skillfully designed and fabricated, were uncovered in the ashes of Pompeii, but no real progress in orthodontics was made between Etruscan times and the middle of the last century. The old world, it seems, contented itself with developing philosophy and psychoanalysis, leaving it to the brash newcomers on the other side of the Atlantic to perfect the flush toilet, the Rotary (club), the hamburger, and modern orthodontics.

Of course, it was no accident that Kingsley and Farrar began to fashion a brand new cosmetic/health specialty when they did and where they did. They combined two unique American ingredients: a gift and a passion for mechanics with a national interest—obsession would, perhaps, be too strong a word—in good grooming. The profession that emerged from this happy connection now includes more than 4,000 specialist members of the American Association of Orthodontists and no one knows exactly how many general practitioners who offer some part time orthodontic care. (There are approximately 104,000 dentists all told in the United States.)

How many Americans begin orthodontic therapy each year? We can't be sure. Neither the American Dental Association nor the American Association of Orthodontists has compiled any statistics on the matter. We can make an educated guess, however. Counting 100 new patients per specialist, which wouldn't be too far from the mark, we arrive at a figure of 400,000 per annum. Since, according to epidemiological (public health) surveys which we *do* have, one out of every five children suffers from a *severe* malocclusion, we can estimate what the acute need is. There are some 4,000,000 live births in America every year. That would mean 800,000 children, or twice as many as the specialists are now treating would derive great benefit from orthodontic care. This doesn't even include the less critical, non-handicapping cases. Are general practitioners taking up the slack? Perhaps. But no one knows the answer to that question either. It would appear, though, that as payment plans become more readily obtainable, demand will outstrip means of health care delivery. Improved techniques and wider use of auxiliary personnel—assistants—are two possible ways of solving the problem. Strong trends for utilization of both methods are already well under way.

Most of the present day patients are children, under 16 years of age. But there is no age limit for the effectiveness of orthodontics. For most, the course of treatment lasts roughly two years. Usually, appliances are cemented in place, exposing their unhappy possessor to taunts of "tinsel teeth" or "metal mouth." The stigma of the braces however is often less humiliating than the original condition and can thus be borne stoically.

Whether the appliances are worn with philosophic resignation or stubbornly resisted can be a matter of crucial importance. Frequently, the braces just won't work unless the patient follows directions with some approximation of good faith. It's his job to hook up the various kinds of elastic force that are designed to ease the teeth from unhealthy, unsightly positions to places where they will be able to resist disease and look good while doing it. All too often even the most sophisticated appliance with an unwilling patient, is, as the lyric tells us, like a ship without a rudder, like a boat without a sail. Without the patient's cooperation even the cleverest of contraptions is all dressed up with no place to go.

Chapter Two

MALOCCLUSION, WHAT IS IT?

We may live without poetry, music and art;
We may live without conscience and live without heart;
We may live without friends; we may live without books;
But civilized man cannot live without cooks . . .
He may live without books—what is knowledge but grieving?
He may live without hope,—what is hope but deceiving?
He may live without love,—what is passion but pining?
But where is the man that can live without dining?

Edward Robert Bulwer Lytton, Lucile

If your physician is going to be able to help you—prescribe the right medicine, tell you whether to go to bed or to run around the block—first he has to determine if you've got that funny little rash on your chest from eating strawberries or because you're coming down with measles. He has to make a decision. He has to establish a diagnosis. Some diseases are not easily classified. Mental illness, for example, is hard to pin down. A few investigators, like Thomas Szasz, are going so far as to call it a myth.

Well, irregularities of the teeth are certainly not a myth. They are right there, for all to see, just as plain as the nose on your face, so to speak. But are crooked teeth a disease? If not, what are they? Must they be straightened, for health reasons, or to preserve the joy of dining that Bulwer Lytton prized so highly? Or are we really dealing exclusively with problems of appearance? Because, after all, even a person who has suffered the ultimate calamity and lost all of his teeth can still get through the meal with dentures. Let's pause briefly to talk about orthodontic diagnosis.

At the turn of the century, Edward Angle began to popularize the term malocclusion. By this he meant teeth of one jaw meeting — occluding with — the other jaw improperly. In a Class I occlusion, the teeth *do* meet properly. (See figure 1.) But if they are crooked or spaced, it's a Class I *mal*occlusion, something of a contradiction in terms, but Angle had a strong personality and managed to get his ideas accepted even if they were a little confusing. In a Class II malocclusion, the upper teeth stick out. In a Class III malocclusion the lower teeth are too prominent. Many times only teeth are involved. If so, the prognosis is good. But if parts of the upper jaw itself are too protrusive in a Class II case or the lower jaw too big in a Class III problem, the deformity is serious and hard to treat. If *too* much mis-matching of jaws is involved, it might be necessary to consider correction by surgical orthodontics, which is quicker and more dramatic than standard treatment. Of course, it is also a far more serious undertaking. The Class II cases, the familiar Bugs Bunny type, are by far the most frequently encountered. It has been estimated that Class III cases occur only about 5% of the time. This is the "undershot" jaw, the type worn with such dash and verve by the royal Hapsburg House of Europe. (See figures 2-4.)

Is that all? Not quite. What does your dentist mean, for instance, when he starts talking about "bite"? Well, in the Class II or Class III kinds of malocclusion, the "bite" is out of alignment either forwards or backwards, that is on the horizontal plane. In a Class III case the lower anterior teeth bite in front of the uppers, not the other way around which is the normal pattern. This is called an anterior cross bite. Teeth on the side, the cheek teeth, can also bite across from where they are supposed to, leading to various possibilities of cross bite. (See fig. 4.)

In the vertical plane, things can go wrong in a couple of ways. With an open bite, the front teeth don't meet at all. Often such a problem is associated with tongue or finger sucking habits and it often looks as though the habit caused the open bite. On the other hand, in instances where the upper teeth come down too far and cover the lower teeth when the back teeth are meeting, it almost seems too bad there hadn't been a habit of some kind to open things up a bit. With all these possibilities for teeth to stray from an ideal pattern, it isn't surprising that some studies have put the incidence of malocclusion as high as 95%. In Chapter 1, it was mentioned that 20% of American children suffered from handicapping dental deformities, a high figure, but far less than 95%. Why such a big difference? Clearly, because some malocclusions constitute serious liabilities and others just do not. How is one to tell what conditions ought to be treated and which ones can safely be left alone?

Dental health is clearly threatened by traumatic crossbites. In cases where teeth occlude so badly that one or more of them may quite literally be knocked right out of the mouth, something ought to be done. Steep over-bite can also be troublesome. It often, but not always, leads to gum troubles in later life. Serious crowding can also cause gingival disease and may increase the likelihood of cavities. Grossly protruding (buck) teeth are more vulnerable to fracture than teeth that are safely behind the lips. Cases of cleft palate, which occur once in every 700 births, also need orthodontic care. But this developmental defect, caused by failure of parts of the upper jaw to meet properly, must be dealt with by a medical team including surgeons, speech therapists, and sometimes psychologists, as well as dentists.

Most of the other kinds of malocclusion, the rotated teeth, the spaced teeth, the moderate protrusions, do not pose any kind of risk for continuing physical well being.

If there aren't any solid medical reasons for correcting these defects, does it really make any sense to spend so much time, money, and effort in pushing around the teeth of America's youth? That all embracing question will be examined in the next chapter.

Chapter Three

THE EMOTIONAL IMPORTANCE OF TEETH

> A little while ago it was your teeth that were to blame for everything. And now, after you have gone and had tin-types taken of your teeth, showing them riding in little automobiles or digging in the sand, some more specialists come along and discover that, after all, it is your glands that are the secret of your mental, moral, and physical well being.
>
> Robert Benchley, "The new bone-dust theory of behavior — Is your elbow all it should be?" *Chips off the old Benchley*.[1]

When Benchley, the amiable Harvard essayist with a captivating, straight-toothed smile, was asked, in his college days, to "discuss the arbitration of the international fisheries problem in respect to hatcheries protocol and dragnet and trawl procedure as it affects (a) the point of view of the United States, and (b) the point of view of Great Britain," he stared thoughtfully at his examination booklet for a long time. Finally, he wrote, "I know nothing about the point of view of Great Britain in the arbitration of the international fisheries problem, and nothing about the point of view of the United States. Therefore I shall discuss the question from the point of view of the fish." The instructor laughed uproariously and flunked Benchley in the course.

We have spent some time examining what malocclusion looks like to orthodontists. We shall continue to outline what parents need to know about dental deformities. But there is another participant who plays a role, however small. The patient. All too often, like the fish, or like the little boy whose mother is buying him a suit, he tends to be ignored. In *How To Be a Jewish Mother,* Dan Greenberg records the parent's inquiry, *to the salesman,* "How does it feel in the crotch?"[2] Let's take a moment to ask what the patient, who may feel like a fish with tight pants, thinks about all this.

There isn't going to be any single, unanimous opinion. Ali McGraw, the actress, stoutly refuses to have her severely-rotated upper incisors straightened. She likes them that way. The same defect for an average teen-ager somewhere in Suburbia or for Billy Graham might be unbearable. Sandy Dennis, like Gene Tierney before her as some mature readers and fans of the late show may remember, were afflicted with moderately pronounced Class II protrusions. Their acting careers don't seem to have been adversely affected. And Eleanor Roosevelt was burdened by a classical kind of double protrusion of both jaws, but she managed to keep going nicely all the same, in spite of it. The late First Lady's malocclusion didn't prevent her from radiating charm, energy and enthusiasm at a rate that would have forced lesser women to take frequent naps or sent them to an early grave.

For many people, much smaller defects would be crippling. In the United States, enormous valuation is placed on appearance, particularly by teenagers. One psychiatrist remarks, "At no other time in life are physical beauty and prowess such critical standards of one's popularity and success."[3] The teenagers, who make up the bulk of the orthodontic population, tend to be highly concerned with the real or imagined stigma that a malocclusion symbolizes. In a nation where face-lifting, hair reweaving and replantation, and nose and breast surgery have become acceptable strategies in the dating game, orthodontic treatment seems almost commonplace in comparison.

Teenagers have good reason to pay so much attention to their appearance. Recent psychological studies by Berscheid and Walster have confirmed that "beauty not only has a more important impact on our lives than we previously suspected but its influence may begin startlingly early." To a surprisingly large extent, most of us judge other people by how they look. "Attractiveness," continue Berscheid and Walster, is the "standard by which we form our first impressions" [4] of our fellows.

Likewise, the opinion of what sociologists call "significant others" determines what kind of an image we form of ourselves. One well-known study, described by Rosenthal and Jacobson in their book *Pygmalion in the Classroom*, reports that two similar groups of children who have been clearly, but incorrectly, labeled for their teachers as "bright" or "dull" will tend to achieve grades that match the description. Intelligence tests are similarly affected.[5]

If, in a remorseless chain, our appearance controls what others think of us which in turn determines how we regard ourselves, then, obviously, any *change* in how we look can be critically important. Such a notion, that alteration of appearance might have a profound impact on a patient's self-esteem, has attracted the attention not only of psychologists, psychiatrists, and sociologists, but it has also interested plastic surgeons for many years. Possibly because their treatment modifies facial structures so slowly that its effects go unnoticed from day to day—while the results of plastic surgery are immediately apparent, at least as soon as the swelling subsides—orthodontists have to date given little notice to this aspect of their endeavors. But orthodontic treatment can often cause transformations fully as dramatic as anything produced by the surgeon's scalpel. The conclusion is inescapable that questions of what psychiatrists call body image should be considered by orthodontists fully as much as they are already taken into account by plastic surgeons.

Knorr and his co-workers explained to their readers in the *Journal of Plastic and Reconstructive Surgery*[6] that children handicapped by "congenital facial deformity," a category that would embrace many orthodontic patients, live in an environment where:

> Attitudes of overprotection, rejection, guilt, anxiety, and depression surrounding the deformed child are emphasized. The body image concept concerning the face may not develop in children until ages 4 to 5; an informal survey of parents with deformed children indicates that the affected child does not perceive himself as different from other children until this age. The full effect of the deformity may not be felt until the child comes under the influence of peers who may reject, ridicule and alienate the child as some one different. *Developmentally, the impaired self-image proves substantially more disabling than the physical defect.* (emphasis added.)

Armed with the insights and the experience painfully garnered by plastic surgeons and their psychiatric colleagues, orthodontists are now in a position to answer the question, raised earlier, "If there is no compelling medico-dental reason to correct a malocclusion, why bother?" Answer: Because the patient's emotional well-being may require it. How does it feel in the crotch to the little boy himself? Forget the viewpoint of the Great Powers (Mom and Dad). What the fish think about is a serious question after all.

The fish may be quite anxious to do something about their looks. Some years after the completion of orthodontic treatment, one young lady was asked what she had thought about in the beginning. She replied:

> I was becoming extremely self-conscious and over-sensitive about my teeth. My overbite was not extreme

but the snide remarks that classmates used to make (Bucky, etc.) really bothered me. It got to the point I would cover my mouth when I laughed . . . or smiled . . . Of course, I did feel self-conscious while I was wearing the braces . . . I was always very shy. I was afraid of having people laugh at me. Bad teeth make you withdraw a little more into yourself. After having braces, I had more confidence in myself as far as being attractive to other people goes. As long as the physical part was taken care of I could work on personality.

The question of the impact on body image created by changes in appearance is complicated. When the correction is swift, as in plastic reconstruction or surgical orthodontics, a technique which will be discussed in chapter 14, psychological adjustment can sometimes be difficult. Some insecure people use facial deformities as an excuse for their inability to cope with the world. "No one likes me because of my big nose or my buck teeth or my terrible scar. It's not my fault," they seem to say. Removal of the stigma for these patients can be a crippling blow. Some of them may experience such severe shock when they find their emotional problems persist despite the elimination of the blemish that they become psychotic, experience a nervous breakdown. Evidently, the painstaking nature of orthodontic treatment, almost always over twelve months long, gives even the most disturbed personalities time to adjust gradually to a new appearance. There have been no reports of psychotic breaks produced by orthodontic manipulations.

This doesn't mean the change in body image always has completely desirable effects. One stunning young female revealed that, "I've definitely got more friends. I used to be shy . . . I like to smile a lot which I never used to. . . .

I really like the way I look now. I'm glad I got them done. My grades have dropped off because I hang around more with my friends. I get out more."

Generally speaking, though, modifications in body image that flow from orthodontic treatment are favorable. More than is realized, perhaps, orthodontics deals with a part of the body that is highly significant to all of us. Freud and the psychoanalytic school regard it as an erogenous zone, profoundly charged emotionally through life. But especially in infancy where the mouth provides the first, and only, means of expression does it possess great importance. Further, still according to psychoanalytic theory, it plays a vital role in the formation of body image. The teeth themselves are not just tools, primitive accessories to the knife and fork. Symbolically, the psychoanalysts say, the teeth represent virility in men, femininity for women. The loss of a tooth is symbolic castration.

Whatever one may think of this type of reasoning, it seems clear that the mouth and teeth have great importance to everyone. It is not surprising that successful orthodontic treatment is sometimes accompanied by corresponding behavioral changes. In the author's experience, overweight girls have begun diets that they could never manage before their teeth were straightened. "When I came here," said one girl, "I weighed 165 lbs. Just in the course of having my teeth taken care of I started taking care of my body appearance also. There was a great loss of weight, about 35 lbs." She has kept her new figure for over six years.

There may even be a connection between facial appearance and intelligence, as the work of Rosenthal and Jacobson suggested. Indeed, Dr. Langdon Down, when he was physician to the Earlswood Asylum for Idiots near London became convinced that there was a high correlation between dental irregularity and mental retardation. Mental *and* dental, he might have said, when he described the characteristics of the so-called mongoloid type of idiocy, now known after him as Down's syndrome.[7] We realize, of course, today, that there is no invariable connection between mental retardation and crooked incisors but certain unattractive arrangements of teeth *do* seem to give an appearance of dim wittedness. Edgar Bergen realized this when he made his country bumpkin mannikin, Mortimer Snerd, into an orthodontic cripple. Charlie McCarthy, the epitome of wooden wit, was, by contrast, equipped with alluringly regular incisors. Isn't it likely that with good-looking teeth and increased confidence, children might begin to perform better than they did when they felt themselves to be unattractive?

Chapter Four

WORKERS IN THE FIELD: WHO TREATS MALOCCLUSION?

> Monkeys, whenever you look, do it;
> Ali Khan and King Farouk do it;
> Let's do it . . .
>
> Noel Coward and Cole Porter,
> *Let's Do It*

You think your child, or possibly you, yourself, have an orthodontic problem that could be relieved. (You may have sneaked a hasty look at Chapter 2 and decided that you or your offspring fall into Angle Class II but you really don't care about the name of the thing. You wonder if you should have it fixed.) What do you do next? If your family dentist has said nothing about it, don't be afraid to ask him. Perhaps there's a specialist in your area to whom you can be referred. Or, if you know of an orthodontist by reputation, you may wish to consult him directly. That's all right, too. By the way, you don't have to worry about fee-splitting in orthodontics. This practice, which is said to plague other endeavors, never seems to have afflicted orthodontics, perhaps because so far there have been more patients needing help than orthodontists were able to handle readily.

Usually the family dentist isn't going to want to treat an orthodontic defect. He simply hasn't been trained to do so. For many reasons, one of which is an over-crowded curriculum that is now being squeezed into three years from four, most dentists are taught little useful information about orthodontics in their school days. Some hard-bitten observers have commented that another, more cogent, reason is that the orthodontic professors who teach the subject simply don't want to reveal too much.

The specialist teachers retort that their field is too complicated for presentation on an undergraduate level thus echoing the sentiments of Publius Syrus who remarked, "Better be ignorant of a matter than half know it." Whoever is right in this dispute, the fact is that general dentists find it difficult to pick up much information about the rudiments of tooth straightening. Still, a good many have made the effort and are banding together in new organizations of "generalists" who do orthodontics while continuing the regular practice of dentistry. Three such groups are the American Institute of Orthodontics, the International Association of Orthodontists and the American Society for the Study of Orthodontics.

The specialists are represented by the American Association of Orthodontists which tends to look with disfavor on the part-timers. All AAO members must agree to abandon general practice and devote themselves exclusively to their specialty. Jurisdictional disputes between the groups have occasionally become inflamed enough to boil over into the courts. The perplexed parent naturally doesn't want to get entangled in this private battle. He simply yearns for good treatment for his child and, if possible, would like not to have to pay too much for it. Maybe the specialist does know more than the dental jack-of-all-trades, but won't his fee be too high?

There is no simple answer to this question, of course. But before even looking at it, let's see what constitutes a specialist. Nowadays, the only dentist allowed by the American Dental Association to announce to the public that he is a specialist in orthodontics is one who has completed a prescribed post-graduate course in a university of at least two years' duration. There have been a few programs in hospitals and at least one attempt, in California, to offer training to selected under-graduate students so the beginning orthodontists wouldn't be superannuated before they get started in their clinical practice. And, until recently, a system of preceptorship permitted recognized orthodontists to train younger men in their offices. Many such former preceptees belong to the American Association of Orthodontists where other members are all graduates of approved university programs. And only members of the AAO were, until quite recently, eligible to apply for certification by the American Board of Orthodontics, the pinnacle of orthodontic achievement. Such men are board eligible and, after passing the examination, are referred to as diplomates of the ABO.

In addition, one other specialty, pedodontics, takes a particular interest in malocclusions developing in its patients. Dentists who are trained in this area limit their practices to caring for dental ailments of infants and children just as pediatricians deal only with the medical care of young people. Pedodontists are primarily concerned with what they call interceptive orthodontics, hoping by nipping mal-functions in the bud to prevent serious disorders from getting established. Some of them may also wish to treat more serious deformities.

To make matters worse there is at least one major issue dividing various categories of practitioners. The bone of contention (very likely a *jaw* bone of contention) entered the picture with Dr. Angle at the turn of the century. Before his time it had seemed reasonable to pioneer orthodontists, who were more or less feeling their way in the dark (the illuminating beams of X-Rays and electricity had not quite come into the picture) to extract a tooth now and then to make room for the others. Angle came to feel that serious excesses were being committed and, in his seventh edition of *Malocclusion of the Teeth*,[1] categorically condemned extractions for orthodontic purposes. With something like religious fervor, the die-hard proponents of extraction were attacked and virtually driven into hiding. But by 1940 some leading American orthodontists, led by the gallant Charles Tweed of Arizona, riding out of the West, despaired of eliminating all crooked teeth and accompanying facial deformities without, as they put it, "resorting" to the removal of teeth. Sometimes they "resorted" to the extraction of "dental units," as though, somehow, the euphemism would lessen the guilt. A stern task master, Angle had trained his followers well in the pursuit of their private holy grail, a perfect set of 32 perfectly aligned teeth. Any compromise with this arbitrary ideal tended to fill the perpetrator with remorse. But the tide began to turn, the sense of guilt lessened, and the extraction camp came to dominate American orthodontic thought.

Meanwhile, in Europe, notably in Germany, holdouts were still expanding the arch, spreading out the teeth in order to keep them all. In fact, the ashes of the great extraction battle, which sometimes seems to take on aspects of Swift's little-enders crusading against the big-enders, never completely died out. The warm coals of controversy have flickered up lately with non-extractionists gaining courage and the extractionists retreating slightly. Many of the general practitioners who do some orthodontics tend to align themselves with the non-extraction school; most full-time orthodontists, but by no means all, would be classified as frequent "resorters" to extraction, although most of them don't apologize so much any more.

What is the baffled patient or parent to make of all this? If he can draw any comfort from the realization that such debates are the rule, not the exception, he can observe similar confrontations in other medical circles. In psychiatry, behavior modifiers and "insight" psychotherapists glare malevolently at each other across the couches and exchange insults. In cancer control we hear lately that breast removals (extractions?) have been much over-done. Some surgeons are claiming they get as good results by cutting away only the tumor and a little surrounding tissue as do their colleagues who remove the entire breast and the adjacent lymph nodes. There is no sign of a truce in that battle. Ophthalmologists refract the drugged eye, optometrists inspect the pure unsullied pupil. And so it goes. Wherever one looks in medicine, one can find plausible arguments supporting diametrically opposed points of view, often about issues of far graver importance than can ever arise in an orthodontic office. No matter how much or how little lies at stake, the prospective client should certainly get at least one other opinion if he doesn't like what he hears the first time. He should insist on a reasonably full evaluation of the problems anticipated and a description of the factors that have influenced the professional decision one way or the other. Later, we shall examine more closely what kinds of choices are available, just why it is the brooding orthodontist must, like the melancholy Dane, ask himself whether 'tis nobler to extract or not to extract. The issues are not so very complicated that the intelligent and well-informed parent or patient cannot participate in the diagnostic process. The life the patient lives is his own and the only one he has. He has every right to play a significant part in determining what happens to his own teeth, his own face, and his own self image.

Chapter Five

THE DIAGNOSTIC DECISION I: GATHERING INFORMATION

> What chance, it may well be asked, has even the lay Lifeman against the Doctor? The Doctor holds all the cards, and can choose his own way of playing them . . . Many Doctors, of course, use Modern Methodship, which consists in irritating or upsetting the patient by the totally irrelevant diagnostic approach . . . A simple method of making a patient feel a fool . . . If he complains of earache after bathing, examine his plantar surfaces . . .
>
> Stephen Potter, *One-Upmanship*

On your first visit to the orthodontist you may want to learn immediately what's wrong with your teeth, if anything, how long it's going to take to deal with your problem, and, in round numbers, how much it is going to cost. If you have a clear cut kind of disorder, with no puzzling mysteries to unravel, everything may very well be explained without delay. Often, however, the examining dentist may feel he cannot give a responsible opinion without taking various measurements to see what category your "case" falls into. He may want to study a cephalometric x-ray.

Figure 5 is a radiograph of the head taken with a device that insures that patient and machine will always be in the same relative position. Subsequent, or serial, pictures can thus safely be compared without requiring allowance for positional variation. From it measurements can be taken which tell whether or not the upper and lower front teeth are where they belong in the skull or are too far forward or too far back and if so how much. This is important because most orthodontists, and presumably most patients, are thinking carefully nowadays not only about getting the teeth straight but also about leaving them in a position where they'll look best in relation to the nose and chin, their concerned neighbors. In other words no one wants to have his teeth improved at the expense of his face. Two other factors must be considered: (1) will the teeth be healthy where they look best, and (2) will the projected position be stable? When these three objectives can be attained by the same solution, there is no problem. When they cannot, a compromise must be chosen. Finally, the orthodontist and his patients, particularly the older ones, must decide if the anticipated gain is worth the cost in effort, money, or discomfort. Some adults, for example, may not feel they need the exquisite corrections that could be achieved by braces that are cemented in place. They may be willing to settle for a result that is dentally less satisfactory than the orthodontist might envisage but that can be achieved by a removable appliance, something most adults can tolerate. Certainly these wishes should be respected so that in the end patients won't endorse the remark Plutarch reports of Caius Marius, "I see the cure is not worth the pain."

We have said that the cephalometric x-ray reveals whether or not the teeth occupy positions where they "belong." There are two basic considerations that must be taken into account. First, the health and stability question. There appear to be clear guide lines to answer this one. The teeth ought to be well supported by the underlying jaw bones—not pushed out too far into an area normally occupied by cheeks or lips and not leaning too far in toward the tongue's domain. With the aid of the cephalometric x-ray, the health-stability aspect of tooth placement can be more or less objectively answered.

But where should the teeth be in order to allow the lips that are draped around them to assume a harmonious pos-

Diagnostic Decision 1: Gathering Information 27

ture? What *is* a harmonious posture? Probably most people can agree on one thing. The teeth should not be so protrusive as to force the lip and facial muscles to strain when the mouth is closed. Is there one best profile toward which all orthodontic treatment efforts should be aimed? For a long time, orthodontists thought so. The ideal was loosely fashioned on the standard of the Grecian Apollo Belvidere. All over America youthful patients were poured into a thin-lipped Anglo-Saxon mold and emerged after two years of meticulous appliance therapy looking like James Cagney even if they were named Giordano Bruno or Simon Ben David or Amos Brown. Recently, thoughtful orthodontists have begun to question the wisdom of forcing all their young clients into the same Procrustean Bed. They find it useful to contemplate a set of norms that will describe safe upper and lower limits for tooth placement from the standpoint of facial appearance. (Since we are talking about moving the teeth toward or away from the tongue, perhaps these limits could more accurately be named inner or outer.) But now they realize that standards that are appropriate for white Anglo-Saxons are meaningless when applied to Asians or Blacks or even Americans of southern European origin. Orthodontists are coming to understand that if beauty is not in the eye of the beholder it at least varies from person to person and observer to observer. Most Blacks and many Jews and Italians seem to look best with full, rounded dental arches and profiles to match that would be unbecoming to Irish Americans. A few orthodontists are even beginning to entertain the uneasy suspicion that their dedicated efforts of the forties and fifties and early sixties to upright teeth and therefore provide flat profiles for all their patients were tainted with unconscious racism.

We can conclude, then, that the orthodontist remains a reliable, informed expert when a decision must be made as to where the anterior (front) teeth should be placed to put them in the most advantageous position for the preservation of dental health. But in determining where to put teeth so as to influence facial contours—to a large extent lip posture reflects tooth position—parents and patients are at least as well equipped to cast a vote as the doctor, and probably more so. After all they know what they like and they have to live with the result. On this issue, at least, patients and parents should make every effort to resist what Potter has called "the natural one-upness of doctors."

The orthodontist may also want to see either a series of individual dental x-rays or one of the new panoramic films which record all the teeth in one long, easy to take picture. These reveal the whereabouts and characteristics of the unerupted teeth still hidden in the jawbones. It is important to know where they are and if they're well formed and headed in the right direction. Sometimes they may be missing entirely. It could be at best embarrassing and at worst disastrous not to find this out in advance.

The orthodontist will need, sooner, or later, plaster models of the teeth. These are taken by having the patient bite into a kind of jello twice, once for each jaw. The procedure is not terribly unpleasant, but people who gag easily might do well to avoid the meal preceding the visit for which impressions are planned. (With the slow, but inevitable acquisition by orthodontists of psychological sophistication, most of the unsettling features of treatment will be attenuated if not entirely eliminated. This topic is treated in somewhat greater detail in Chapter 12.)

The plaster, of course, comes later. It is poured into the "jello," not the mouth. From the resulting models, the orthodontist can make accurate measurements that would be obtained with difficulty on the living patient. Also, these

Diagnostic Decision 1: Gathering Information

models can readily be turned upside down or sideways or inspected carefully from the rear, all of which feats are performed awkwardly on the client himself. In addition, the dentist will probably want to take photographs of the face and teeth. These can not only be measured but are especially useful to demonstrate before and after changes. All of this material, which constitutes a record of the original malocclusion, will help in deciding what's to be done, if anything. In case the condition is unusual, the records can easily be transported to meetings where advice can be obtained from colleagues. Finally, these studies will be useful as a record—hence the name—of the original problem. From time to time he can check against them to see if the anticipated rate of progress is being maintained. At this writing fees for these diagnostic services might range between $45 and $120.

After all the information has been assembled, studied, and digested, the orthodontist may wish to confer with the patient and parents. His objectives may not coincide with those of his client. If there is a stigma associated with crooked teeth, for some children there may be an even greater stigma attached to the braces. On the other hand it is said that in some affluent areas the wearing of appliances is considered to be a desirable sign of status. We should bear in mind that the original malocclusion is handicapping only to the extent that it is perceived as a liability by the patient. This perception is subject not only to individual variation but also to fluctuation between cultures and sub-cultures. When a group of African students was sipping soft drinks on a suburban veranda a few years ago, the hostess excused herself to take the family dog to the veterinarian. The Africans looked puzzled at the explanation. She repeated her description of Fido's proposed checkup. It finally dawned on the visitors that this woman was actually going to spend time, money, and effort on medical care for a household *pet*. Where they live, doctors are not always available for *people*. In some places orthodontic treatment, like a manicure for a cat, would be regarded as frivolous.

Chapter Six

THE DIAGNOSTIC DECISION 2: TO EXTRACT OR NOT TO EXTRACT

> Dente lupus, cornu taurus petit.
> (The wolf attacks with his teeth,
> the bull with his horns.)
>
> Horace, *Satires*, II, 1, 52.

Mankind's most stirring drama, his evolution from simian ancestors, began almost three million years ago somewhere in the grassy savannas of East Africa. One scene from this long-run production is played today in an unlikely setting, the friendly, neighborhood dental office. Every schoolboy knows that the essential difference between man and both his primate relatives and proto-human forebears is the enormous enlargement of the brain case which has permitted the simultaneous development of nuclear physics and rock and roll music. What is not so generally realized is that this growth of intellectual capacity has been accomplished at the expense of the face. As the cranium advances, the dentition retreats. (See figure 6a.) If the outline of a modern mandible were superimposed on the Mauer jaw-bone, the oldest European relic, the ancient fossil would dwarf its contemporary counterpart. (See figure 6b.) Yet the teeth of this emerging human, according to Andre Senet, writing in *Man in Search of his Ancestors*, "were practically identical with those of modern man."[1] No wonder American school children so often have crowded teeth and condemn their parents to pay a hefty orthodontic bill. Their entangled incisors would have had room to spare in the ancestral jaw-bones of *homo habilus* or *homo erectus*.

31

But their own delicate jaws frequently cannot support the same amount of tooth structure that would easily have been accommodated by the robust huntsmen of the prehistoric plains. An orthodontic fee is one of the prices that must be paid for academic achievement (See figures 6c and 6d.)

The evidence for evolutionary shrinkage of the bony support for the dentition would seem to be impressive enough to convince any but the most dedicated believer in special creation. In this light, extraction of teeth is seen as a reasonable remedy for a lack of harmony between parts. Of course, if God created man in his own image without allowing for any subsequent changes, there ought to be no need to tinker with the design. This greatly resembles the view Edward Hartley Angle finally settled on and first proclaimed in 1903, in *Items of Interest,* a pioneering dental periodical. To eliminate confusion and relieve the technician of the wearisome burden of establishing a diagnostic decision, the father of modern orthodontia divulged "a law so plain and so simple that all can understand and apply it. It is that the best balance, the best harmony, the best proportions of the mouth in its relations to the other features requires that there shall be *the full complement of teeth, and that each tooth shall be made to occupy its normal position — normal occlusion."* No longer would it be necessary, he announced, to leave "to the individual judgment of the operator . . . the determination of the requirements . . . in each case." [2]

This was as neat a reversal of field as anything then taking place in football, another activity born and bred in America which, like orthodontia, was enjoying increasing popularity. Only a few years before, in the sixth edition of his magnum opus, *Malocclusion of the Teeth,* Angle had conceded that extractions were required when the jaws were too "small" or when placing the teeth in the "line of occlusion" would "result in marked dental or labial prominence" with the "facial result . . . more unpleasing than if the teeth had been allowed to remain in malpositions." [3]

What made Angle change his mind? Why did he precipitate the great extraction war, a struggle in which occasional skirmishes are still being fought? There is no evidence that Angle opposed therapeutic removal of teeth on fundamentalist religious grounds but it seems likely that he adopted from his aesthetic mentor, Professor E. H. Wuerpel ("one of our foremost teachers of art")[4] some hazy notions of Platonic idealism. In his mind's eye he beheld a perfect set of 32 unravaged teeth, meeting in a perfect "line of occlusion," and sharing in the triumphant unfolding of a perfect face unless "Nature" were "greatly taxed in her normal processes of growth by accident and especially by certain forms of disease which interfere with her delicate work." [5] In other words, the causes of malocclusion were entirely environmental. The task of the orthodontist was, essentially, that of a railroad switchman. He had to get the temporarily derailed train of occlusion back on the track.

There was to be no single standard of facial beauty, but, in Wuerpel's words, "a law for each individual." [6] The professor avowed that "It is because we are conscious of an ideal type to which we belong that we strive to create in our minds and in our persons this type. This is what the Greeks did." Inspired by Wuerpel, Angle embarked on his quest for the perfect face. For a time he persuaded virtually the entire profession to join him. Among the ardent followers was Charles Tweed. But gradually, regretfully, even guiltily, Tweed convinced himself that in spite of Angle's promises that the jaw bones would grow to harmonize with the restored "line of occlusion" some of his most carefully treated cases were relapsing to the original crowding. Other patients looked worse (or in Angle's memorable phrase "more unpleasing") after treatment than before. One probable victim of such iatrogenic (treatment induced) disease was Eleanor Roosevelt, earlier described as stigmatized by bimaxillary protrusion. This may have been caused by an orthodontist declining to remove teeth. Her biographer, Joseph Lash, tells us in *Eleanor and Franklin* that "Jessie* was the prettiest girl in class, and Eleanor, who was gawky, her prominent teeth in braces, *admired her for her loveliness.*"[7] (Emphasis added.) Tweed came to feel that no matter what Angle had said, in some cases he had to order the removal of teeth. Had he, or someone like him, been called in to care for poor young Eleanor, she might have been spared much unhappiness. Curiously, a benign fate finally remedied the early professional oversight. Writing in the *Angle Orthodontist*, a friend, Frances Macgregor, recalled, "Mrs. Roosevelt, whom I knew well, reported in her writings her feelings about being what she called an 'ugly duckling.' She . . . had to struggle long and valiantly before she at last succeeded (overtly at least) in overcoming her feelings of inferiority and shyness . . . During her years as First Lady, caricatures of her were legend—always with large protruding teeth. Although so late in her lifetime, she finally had relief from this. She was in an automobile accident and lost, as I recall, three or four of her front teeth. Following dental restoration she told me with unabashed delight what a fortunate accident it had been, because at last she had straight front teeth."[8]

Whatever their outlook on idealism, modern orthodontists agree that many of their potential patients seem to

---

* Jessica Sloane, a classmate at Roser, who later became the Baroness Emilay de la Grange. With protrusions or without, Roser girls seem to have married well.

Diagnostic Decision 2: To Extract or Not to Extract

have insufficient room for all their teeth. Never mind whether this derives exclusively, as Angle believed, from accident or disease, or from hereditary factors. A great body of research, beginning with the work of the English anatomist, physiologist, and surgeon, John Hunter, in the 18th century, has conclusively demonstrated that the portion of the jaw supporting the anterior teeth does not grow appreciably after children reach the age of six.[9] Thus little relief can be anticipated from growth—jaws just aren't going to develop enough in dimensions that will be useful for tooth straightening purposes.

This means that one of three alternatives must be selected if the needed space is to be obtained orthodontically:

1) The posterior teeth can be moved backward and the front teeth eased slightly forward to create the desired room. There are limits to how much pushing can be done in either direction. Behind, the unerupted second and third molars stand ready to resist too much encroachment on *their* territory and in front the lips, surprisingly strong and muscular when threatened with invasion, will fight back against any attempt to usurp *their* domain. And the orthodontist who pushes anterior teeth too far forward risks creation of the Eleanor Roosevelt syndrome.

2) Space can be obtained by reducing total tooth size. Aristotle allegedly proclaimed that 28 teeth constituted a full set because he never took the trouble to count them. Most people today know that there are supposed to be 32 even if they haven't personally verified this computation. Most people are also aware that often there isn't room for all 32, sometimes not even for 28. Teeth as they erupt at various ages may be squeezed out of the arch and others, especially the last to arrive, the wisdom teeth, may get so seriously stuck that they are said to be impacted. Then

they don't come in at all. To prevent these mishaps, or correct them if they've already occurred, tooth size may be reduced in two ways:

> a) The extraction solution that caused Angle so much anguish may be resorted to. Usually, nowadays, this is done in a balanced way. Four side teeth are usually chosen: one from each quadrant, upper left. upper right, lower left, lower right.
>
> b) Recently another method of cutting down tooth size has been tried out on a wide scale. And that's just how it is done—by *cutting down* the sides of the teeth a little bit at a time in a kind of sand-papering procedure that sounds alarming but doesn't seem to hurt a bit. It's called inter-proximal stripping.[10]

3) The dental arches of both jaws can be gently expanded sideways, toward the cheeks. This technique was exhaustively tested in this country, and all over the world, for that matter, after Angle proclaimed that extractions were biologically, and probably ethically, misguided. Agreeing with Tweed, most American orthodontists have concluded that the results of expansion do not consistently remain stable. The cheeks it appears were too strong a counter force to outward migration of the teeth. When the orthodontist and his patient pushed one way the cheeks pushed back, harder.

One group of dentists, many of them not full time orthodontists, as we have seen, remains unconvinced. They have revived the expansion technique with somewhat modified mechanical devices. They are persuaded as was Angle, that Nature intended all their patients to retain a full complement of teeth and insist that *their* efforts will not collapse. Further, they argue, when extractions are carried out for patients whose facial contours do not require it the lips may drop back *too* far giving the profile an unattractive, excessively concave, prematurely aged look. The extractionists argue back in three general ways:

1) They point to the evolutionary reduction of the face and expansion of the cranium. Modern man no longer needs powerful jaws to rip apart freshly killed game or, in fact, to kill it in the first place. Twentieth century gourmets need to expend little effort to chew their highly refined food. Their small jaws reflect these reduced duties. But the teeth, substantially identical with early man's, find they cannot all fit into their cramped quarters.[11]

2) The question of diet was amplified by Raymond Begg, who, after studying with Angle, returned to his native Australia where he developed a highly effective mechanism to treat malocclusion and simultaneously worked out a compelling theory to account for the high incidence of crowding in contemporary dentitions. Stone age man, Begg said, chewed such highly abrasive foods that his teeth were so worn down, so reduced in size in every dimension, that there was plenty of room for each successive tooth to erupt into the mouth.[12] With our over-civilized diet no such abrasion occurs. The orthodontist has no recourse but to simulate the no longer operative sand papering effect with some artificial sandpaper of his own or to extract four teeth entirely.

3) Ethnically pure stocks, some observers have noted, tend to have relatively uncrowded teeth. Where groups of widely varying backgrounds have mixed genetic input, as in the United States, input for large teeth too often is crossed with coding for a small jaw contributed by a different ancestor. The result of this genetic jumble is the alarming report that 95% of our children have crooked teeth. (More conservative estimates of the occurrence of mal-

occlusion begin with a claim that one of five American children have severe dental deformities.)

As in every medical controversy, no doubt there is merit in both arguments. Probably both extremes ought to be avoided. Wuerpel might have noted that the Romans had a phrase for it: follow the golden mean.

Chapter Seven

FURTHER DIAGNOSTIC ADVENTURES

> Where order in variety we see
> And where, though all things
> differ, all agree
>
> Alexander Pope, *Windsor Forest.*

Nature has a way of trying out everything. In her evolutionary rambles she has experimented with most conceivable life styles, from the amoeba to the dinosaur, from the kangaroo to Tiny Tim. As the plot unfolds, century by century, certain trends, we have seen, slowly become apparent. For *homo sapiens*, the snout recedes as the brain enlarges. Some changes are greeted with joy. Others, like crowded teeth and baldness, are irksome. But good or bad, any given characteristic appears in a wide range of possibilities which shades gradually from one extreme to the other. In any large population representatives of each of these forms will turn up in a random way following what is called a normal distribution. In addition to this individual dispersion there is wide variation between groups. Facial appearance accordingly changes from region to region —no one would have trouble distinguishing *any* Parisian from *any* Australian bushman. Teeth show the same kinds of variation. So, while there is a clear tendency for many people to have crowded dentitions, others will have teeth that are less crowded, some will have teeth that are not crooked at all, and there will even be others whose teeth are spaced.

When this problem arises, if it is unsightly enough, the orthodontist, in consultation one hopes with his clients and the family dentist, has to decide whether to close the spaces or open them up so that replacements standing in for the absent parties can be installed. If all the spaces *can* be closed and if it is reasonable to hope they will stay closed, this is the procedure of choice. No bridges or false teeth will be needed. But closing spaces usually means that teeth must be moved lingually—toward the tongue where there is no assurance they will stay put. (Lloyds of London refuses to write a policy on it.) In some people the tongue is a stubborn bundle of muscles that thrusts persistently where it shouldn't causing trouble like the re-opening of orthodontically closed spaces. Also, transportation of the teeth too far toward the tongue may force the lips to adopt an unpleasant caved in appearance. A safe course must be elected between the Scylla of depending on false teeth and the Charybdis of "dishing in" the profile. The dilemma is greater when teeth are missing. No one knows why an otherwise normal jaw grows to maturity minus one or more teeth. Physical anthropologists might be willing to guess, though, that such failures are tentative signs of evolutionary adjustment. If modern man has jaws that are tiny in comparison with humanoid ancestors but teeth that are more or less unchanged in size, one way for Nature to arrange a renewed balance would be to reduce the number of teeth, to lower the human dental formula. This may be what is happening. Not infrequently second bicuspids, lateral incisors, and third molars either fail completely to begin formation or are badly stunted in size or shape.

More rarely other teeth neglect to make an appearance at the appointed place and time. When upper lateral incisors, the teeth next to the ones on the center line, are dwarfed in size, or "peg-shaped" they look like a dental version of Long John Silver's wooden leg. In these cases one might imagine that Nature after deciding to scratch the entry entirely had second thoughts and, grudgingly, permitted the emergence of a reasonable facsimile. The orthodontist must predict whether or not this ill-favored tooth, when properly positioned, will look good enough to be retained as is, will eventually pass muster but only if capped, or will best contribute to the over-all appearance of the mouth by making a graceful and permanent exit. If extractions are being considered as a part of the treatment plan, whenever possible the weakest teeth, abandoning all thought of self, should be allowed to make the final sacrifice for the common good.

All other things being equal, certain side teeth, the bicuspids, work out best as choices for extraction. But, substitutions can sometimes be made. Peg-shaped laterals should be sacrificed if it is anticipated that the next teeth in line, the cuspids, can be persuaded to take their place and will not look too obtrusive masquerading through life as lateral incisors. Varying amounts of reshaping, sometimes even capping, are required to bring off this deception since the cuspid tooth is strong, squat, and sturdy while the lateral is slight and shapely. Of course, if the laterals or other teeth are missing, the choice of teeth to be extracted has been pre-determined by a higher power. In cases where large cavities or other disasters make long term retention of a tooth dubious, careful thought must be given to awarding it the noble role of sacrificial lamb. When this is done, it is usually wise to "balance" the extractions by selecting the same or quite similar teeth from each of the four quadrants of the mouth. In most instances, extractions must be carried out in this evenhanded manner, one tooth from each of the four corners of the jaws, to preserve or make possible the correct intermeshing of upper teeth with lower. If teeth are removed from one jaw and not the other an unhealthy imbalance between them is likely to be created and if teeth are extracted from one side and not the other, the dentition will tend to drift sideways and make not only itself but also the face look lopsided. But what if the estimated space requirement per quadrant is only half a tooth or less? Must a whole tooth be sacrificed from each of the four corners? Usually, yes. Angle was certainly right when he described the "anterior component of force" which propels back teeth forward throughout life. This is why, Begg later said, teeth which are worn down in size because of harsh diet—Begg referred to the process as attritional occlusion—still kept contact with their neighbors. They are, like good football linemen, constantly driving forward. So by the time treatment is finished and allowance is made for the possible eruption of third molars later on, all of that room may eventually prove useful. But if the orthodontist is convinced he really doesn't need as much space as four teeth would provide, he has two choices. If he wants just a little added working area, he might try to filch it by gentle expansion and hope for the best. Or he could plan on imitating Begg's natural process of attritional occlusion with some artificial attrition created by his sandpapering device referred to earlier.

Since all things differ, as the poet said, it is not surprising that in human dentitions not only do teeth fail to appear from time to time but occasionally they do just the opposite: they occur in over-abundance. When this happens, when supernumeraries are present, no soul searching is required. The extra teeth are simply extracted unless they lie in such difficult positions that their removal would require too troublesome an operation. Rarely, an extra tooth is such an exact replica of a normal member of the dental team that the two can't be told apart. In such a case, the tooth in the least favorable location can be eliminated. Another unusual occurrence is twinning. The extra tooth may be physically joined to its mate like a Siamese twin. Here the orthodontist must determine whether or not he can include this cumbersome fellow in the extraction plan and thus be rid of him. If it's a front tooth whose absence may be embarrassing later on, he may try to slim it down by patient sanding.

So far we've described most of the physical deviations from a theoretical ideal that the orthodontist sees. Orthodontists agree on how to deal with the majority of these problems except crowding. Moving along to the area of behavior, we see to our dismay that the battle lines have been redrawn and that the smoke of battle clouds this modern confrontation as thickly as it ever enveloped Angle and his extractionist foes. What behavior? What controversy? Thumb sucking, of course.

For some, it is a nasty habit to be broken at all costs. For others it is merely a product of faulty learning that can be unlearned by application of the proper techniques. And for still others it is a symptom of deep-seated yearnings, tied up with basic sexual instincts, and, all in all, a business that had better be approached with the greatest care, skill, and delicacy. The conscientious parent who had, perhaps, begun to sort out his feelings on the extraction issue and decided what position to take will be forgiven if he sighs, "My God, this is where I came in. Total confusion!"

What is this debate all about? It depends on the point of view. Persistent and intense thumb or finger sucking will unquestionably displace teeth. Applied diligently enough and long enough, the child's digit works just like an orthodontic appliance, only in the wrong direction. The effects of finger sucking on baby teeth are probably transient. That is, no permanent structures are likely to be seriously affected by this type of pressure applied to baby teeth. But if the habit continues after the age of seven, when grown up teeth first join the scene, it can open up glaring and lasting spaces. From a mechanical point of view the process ought to be stopped immediately. And that's exactly what dedicated dentists have been trying to do for the last seventy years. (Not the same fellows, of course; they do it in relays.) Labelling the activity "pernicious" or "noxious" they have, with the best of intentions, tried to "break" it by a variety of ingenious devices. Bristly, pointy "hayrakes" have been cemented into mouths to keep the offending finger out; thumbs have been strapped to fingers; elbows immobilized; arms themselves pinioned by near straitjackets; and various foul tasting potions painted on youthful thumbs—all to break the habit. The over-all success of this approach is debatable but the effort proceeds despite formidable resistance from many psychiatrists. "Slow down," they have said, "a malocclusion of the mind is more serious than a malocclusion of the teeth." And that, they have explained, was exactly what would result from ill-advised efforts to deprive a child of the emotional support he derived from a sucking habit. (Try to imagine Linus with his beloved blanket ripped forever from his tender hands. The mind boggles.) Prevent children from obtaining this needed relief, psychoanalytically oriented psychiatrists have said, and they will develop more serious problems which may not be so easily detected. Sophisticated dentists and orthodontists have heeded the warning and the vogue for sharp "hay rakes" has subsided although it has certainly not disappeared. When they are used nowadays they ought to be gentle and rounded like the rolling hills of England not craggy and punishing like the Alps since a recent study has shown that one version of the device is about as effective as the other. In defending use of "hay rakes," advocates point out that parents are quite content with them. This neatly side-steps the possibility that the wishes and needs of parents and children may not always coincide. Witness the distressing frequency of child abuse cases. Certainly forceful restraint of a habit is not the same thing as child beating; but it could be a disguised and diluted shadow of it.

This cautious insight harmonizes with the dynamic nature of psychoanalytic theory which views sucking as a surface symptom of unconscious conflict or need. This behavior, often accompanied by the stroking of a blanket, a "transitional object," is appropriate for certain stages of emotional maturation. Prolonged beyond the proper developmental stage, sucking indicates psychological problems and should be handled with respect and skill. "Nonsense!" behaviorists respond. "The kid has just learned a bad habit and by proper techniques we can show him how to unlearn it without leaving any undesirable side effects whatever."

The behaviorist movement which in relatively recent times has energetically challenged the entrenched psychoanalysts not only in orthodontics but also across a wide spectrum of activities, was founded in America in the 1920's by J. B. Watson who built on the pioneering work of the Russian Pavlov. After a brief period of popularity, behaviorism fell into disrepute until it was revived not long ago by B.F. Skinner's efficient version called operant conditioning and its therapeutic spin-off, behavior modification. Behaviorists either reject the notion of unconscious conflict or consider it to be of no importance. They don't worry about another symptom replacing a "deconditioned" thumb or finger habit. As if it didn't have enough trouble with its durable extraction war, orthodontics now must stand by helplessly as psychotherapy's private battle spills over into dental territory. But even though orthodontic journals print articles that take sides in the controversy between behavior modification and psychoanalysis, there is little evidence that many orthodontists are paying much attention to this new rhubarb in their midst.

Generally, the debate is academic so it doesn't matter that the audience is small. Most children who seem to be irrevocably committed to a finger sucking habit manage to give it up before too much damage has been done. Only a small percentage of parents have to make the painful decision whether to have their child's thumb psychoanalyzed or desensitized by behavior modification. In the rare instances in which the habit is still present when orthodontic treatment begins, it almost always fades away as the braces get cemented into place. Perhaps the parent who finds his child's habit excessively annoying ought to ask himself, "Why is it bothering *me* so much?"

Chapter Eight

FINAL DIAGNOSTIC ADVENTURES—
THE DOCTOR'S DILEMMA

> To blow and swallow at the same time is not easy.
>
> Plautus, *Mostellaria*,
> III, ii, 104.

Finger sucking habits probably arouse vague feelings of guilt in certain parents. An uneasy, largely unconscious realization that the rhythmic, soothing sucking behavior has powerful sexual connotations can be quite upsetting to some adults. Occasionally, in fact, the hidden meaning of the habit becomes clear when sucking patterns are combined with obvious masturbation. With our double heritage of Puritan and Roman Catholic morality, no wonder some adults are angered by such activity. By God, *they* weren't allowed to carry on like that when *they* were children. This may account, at least in part, for the enthusiastic use by some dentists and parents of habit-breaking devices with their thinly disguised punitive features.

In the early days of orthodontics in this country, when Angle and his school were convinced that Nature had a plan for every dentition, it seemed obvious that all malocclusions had to have a specific cause in the environment. Suspicion fell on other habits like nail-biting, pencil-chewing, and lip-biting. Such things are no longer considered to be of any great significance.

Bruxism, which is the grinding or clenching of teeth, can wear down the biting surfaces and transmit unhealthy stress to gums and bone. It may play a small role in the establishment of some disorders but probably not a large one. Not long ago one researcher suggested that everyone has had things inside out all these years—that malocclusion caused bruxism and not vice versa and that nervous tension had nothing to do with it. This seems unlikely.

Mouth breathing, which Angle described as the "most potent, constant, and varied . . . of all the various causes of malocclusion" [1] was recently characterized by a leading authority as "more of an associated . . . factor" and not a "primary causative factor" in the production of malocclusion.[2] Because of this de-emphasis of mouth breathing as a villain in causing crooked teeth, orthodontists are now far less likely than they used to be to order the removal of tonsils and adenoids. Angle and his followers had believed that an overgrowth of these mucous pads at the base of the throat interfered with airways and forced unhappy children to gasp for life-giving ozone with lips permanently agape. At the same time physicians have come to realize that tonsils and adenoids can play a big part in combating infection. So *they* are suggesting fewer operations. This releases the hospital beds needed for orthodontists who suffer nervous breakdowns because they can't decide whether or not to extract teeth or what do about thumb-sucking.

Despite the uncertainty about the psychological implications of finger habits, at least they have the virtue of clear visibility. Parents can recognize them and draft a plan of action. Usually, as we have said, the best action is none at all. Parents should attempt to master any personal feelings of revulsion and allow the habit to melt away in the normal course of development. Unfortunately, there is one habit whose apparent importance has not diminished with changing ideas about the etiology of malocclusion, which is frequently difficult to detect, and which is not likely to disappear of its own accord as the child matures. This stubborn rogue has adopted various aliases: to speech therapists it is tongue thrust, to orthdontists it is abnormal swallowing reflex, and to physiologists it is aberrant deglutition (the same thing in Latin.) Long perplexed by unexpected and inexplicable failures in mechanical treatment, orthodontists now suspect that sneaky tongue activity may be pushing teeth one way just as hard as they push in the other direction.

Unhappily, scientific understanding of reverse swallowing (yet another term) is scarcely more advanced than efforts to describe it with one, simple name. In dealing with the behavior, or misbehavior, of the tongue, dental scientists and their allies have gotten about as far as chickens crossing the road. When they (the scientists, not the chickens) examine a child whose upper front teeth do not meet the lower front teeth in closure—an open bite—they have no idea whether the tongue darts continuously into the space because it is so tantalizingly there or if the space was created by the tongue to begin with. No one is really sure which came first, the chicken, the tongue, the space, or the egg. And since the cause of open bites is uncertain, the correct course of treatment must be equally unclear. If the script is based on a muscle-bound tongue strong-arming innocent teeth apart, it makes sense to rehabilitate the tongue first and deal with teeth later. When this approach is tried, primary treatment is entrusted to the speech therapist. But if a curious tongue is simply slipping into a pre-existing space because it cannot resist temptation, then the malocclusion should be eliminated first in the hope that the wandering tongue will thereupon proceed to take care of itself.

Until recently orthodontists didn't trouble themselves excessively with trying to make this chicken and egg decision. But some of them began to notice some 15 or 20 years ago that a few cases, no matter how well managed, seemed either to resist treatment or, if initially responsive, tended to relapse inexorably. It had generally been assumed that the teeth and dental arches existed in a kind of no-man's land mid-way between the opposing muscular forces of lips and cheeks on one side and the tongue on the other. Generally, these opposing powers lived in harmony but from time to time one of them ran amok pushing teeth aside en route. Recent evidence suggests that the tongue is the more powerful of the two systems. In the usual course of events, it disdains to exert its strength. In normal swallowing, for example, the teeth of the two jaws come gently together and the tongue rests passively against the roof of the mouth or the backs of the front teeth. But in reverse swallowing, the tongue is thrust vigourously between the teeth in conjunction with a hearty contraction of the muscles around the mouth. How come? No one is altogether sure about this, either. According to one scenario, normal swallowing will flow right along with good healthy mother's milk. If early feeding has been somehow inadequate, the child will develop tongue thrusting in compensation. Or, another theory goes, when milk has poured *too* freely from a poorly designed artificial nipple, the child learns aberrant swallowing patterns to save himself from drowning. Whatever their origin, swallowing patterns are reflex in nature and difficult to retrain, sometimes resisting the best joint efforts of speech therapists and orthodontists.

Close examination has revealed that a number of tongue thrust patterns can be isolated. If movement is forward, an open bite between anterior teeth can be expected. If, as sometimes, happens, the tongue roams sideways, more complicated and more elusive problems result: the bite can be adversely affected in a variety of ways. Sometimes a partial open bite and sometimes a partial closed bite can be caused by a lateral tongue thrust. Either one can be difficult to diagnose and just as hard to treat. But even though this discovery seemed at first to add complications it also offered promise of better things to come. Orthodontists would not henceforth have to assume total responsibility for all malocclusions. They could send some of their most recalcitrant tongue-thrusting problems to speech therapists. Some even hoped that when the tongue had been retrained, malplaced teeth, urged along by lip pressure acting like a sheep dog nipping at errant lambs, would glide voluntarily back to their assigned positions. Also, certain relapses could be forestalled by proper attention to tongue control.

Unfortunately, the high hopes of speech therapists and orthodontists have not yet been realized. A few tongue-thrusting problems seem to respond well to treatment, others do not. Similarly, the great expectations entertained by speech therapists that orthodontists could cure some of *their* knottiest problems have not yet come to pass. There is little likelihood that they ever will since the role played by teeth in normal speech is not great. The late Ernie Hixon, a level-headed dental scientist who will be sorely missed, remarked that "Teeth . . . facilitate but are not essential in the articulation of a few labiolingual and linguodental [sounds]."[3] If an orthodontist can manage to correct an open bite he may contribute to improved speech. Reasonable contact of upper and lower anterior teeth is required in the production of the sibilants (f, s, and z) so important to the career of the budding tragic actor. Edwin Booth would have looked pretty silly trying to hiss, "Out damned spot!" through gaping incisors. He might have wound up stammering "Out damned pot!" and cut short his career by 50 years.

Hixon attacked another aspect of conventional wisdom regarding the importance of teeth. "From the standpoint of digestion," he said, "teeth are a convenience . . . but not a necessity for survival." Here, too, only an open bite is handicapping: it limits chewing efficiency. Every other so-called malocclusion can contribute as much to metabolic performance as a perfect set of teeth. (It is true that crowded teeth increase the likelihood of decay and possibly, but not certainly, they hasten the onset of gum disease.) Indeed, Ernie pointed out, total loss of teeth didn't prevent one Mesa Verde Indian from surviving until 130, the last seventy years with no dentition at all. Since this native American did all of his dining more than 700 years ago, he had to do it without the aid of orthodontic technology and he appears to have done it very well. Unlike some of his stuffier colleagues, Ernie realized that what orthodontists refer to as "malocclusion" was really "biologically normal genetic variation." In other words, even the most unattractive dental irregularities are merely extreme entries on a normal curve. Since orthodontic treatment has little survival value but is "highly desirable socially," to quote Ernie once more, it is important that the orthodontist concoct a plan of action that will not only straighten teeth but will also leave the face looking as attractive as possible.[4] This is sometimes difficult since the two objectives do not always harmonize. It is frequently advisable, in order to create sufficient room for all the teeth, to remove some, as we have seen. When this is done, it is almost certain that the front teeth will drop back to a greater or lesser extent in the direction of the extraction spaces. Usually this is desirable. Most candidates for orthodontic treatment not only have crowded dentitions but look as though they had absent-mindedly got a golf ball stuck between their lips and teeth. To put it another way, they find it difficult to keep their mouths shut even when they're not saying anything. In such cases dental and cosmetic requirements coincide. By extracting some teeth it is possible for the orthodontist to straighten the remaining ones and permit the lips to retreat into a comfortable and beguiling posture. But sometimes lips are already far enough or even too far back with respect to nose and chin and yet teeth are jumbled. Extractions would improve the crowding and worsen facial appearance. What to do?

Orthodontists have certain secondary positions they can seek out. Usually the teeth of choice for extractions are the first bicuspids—the fourth tooth from the center—because they are conveniently close to the area where space is needed but not so close that their absence will be noticed when all the teeth have been arranged in order and are touching one another. By going back a little further in the mouth and extracting second bicuspids orthodontists can prevent the front teeth from slipping too far toward the tongue. They can use some of the space for straightening purposes in the front of the mouth and allow the rest to be filled in by back teeth sliding forward. By skillful management of forces, orthodontists try to obtain just enough room to unravel jumbled teeth and none at all for excessive retraction of lips which usually, but not always, follow the lead of anterior teeth.

Sometimes this compromise isn't good enough. The lower front teeth, for example, may be set well back behind a prominent chin. To make matters worse the patient may have a large nose. To correct crowding it may be essential to extract. But to mask the large chin it may be essential to keep all the teeth and, in fact, push the front ones forward. With extractions teeth will straighten but facial appearance will deteriorate. By attempting treatment without extractions, orthodontists may be able to preserve or even improve facial contours but the likelihood of dental collapse later on will be great. There may be no perfect answer to such dilemmas. In some cases it might be best to extract, making every effort to incline the front teeth forward. In others it might be best to keep all the teeth and plan on holding them with some kind of retaining device in corrected, but strained positions, for a long time if not throughout life. In still other cases, stripping may offer a way out.

Bernard Shaw's Sir Colenso Ridgeon faced a problem of quite a different order. Possessing only enough life sustaining medicine for one, he had to decide which dying patient to save, a kindly, bumbling, ineffectual friend or a gifted young painter who was a thorough scoundrel. The question of whether or not to remove teeth from a crowded dentition is not so serious as that. "Tis not so deep a well," as Mercutio said, "nor so wide as a church-door; but 'tis enough, 'twill serve." It is the most disturbing dilemma orthodontists have.

Chapter Nine

DENTAL DATA

>The tooth, the whole tooth, and nothing but the tooth.
>   Robert Benchley.

Stephen Leacock's comic hero, Lord Ronald, one thoroughly confusing day, "flung himself upon his horse and rode madly off in all directions." In order to deal straightaway with a few of the significant issues that affect orthodontic practice, we may seem to have galloped as quickly from Aristotle to Helena Rubinstein. With this intoxicating exploration bravely begun, perhaps it would be prudent to pause to get our bearings and touch lightly on a few fundamentals before pushing on to a further shore. Those readers sufficiently familiar with the essentials of dental anatomy can avoid the detour by turning to Chapter 10.

The teeth are specialized organs designed for eating and fighting and are formed from the same embryonic tissue that produces nails and hair. In man there are twenty baby or deciduous teeth, ten upper and ten lower. These begin to take shape in the jaws before birth. The first to appear in the mouth are the lower central incisors, which erupt at about the age of six months. The teeth are housed in two jaw bones, the maxillae. The upper is referred to simply as the maxilla and the lower is called (rarely) the inferior maxilla or (usually) the mandible. Firmly joined to the skull, the superior maxilla cannot be moved. But it is not entirely monolithic. At birth there are not only two maxillae, left and right, which grow together to form the roof of the mouth, the hard palate, but also two anterior segments, the pre-maxillae which also come together in the mid-line. Even though these sections do not become fully joined until about 17 years of age, they should be reasonably well approximated at birth, separated only by thin belts of soft tissue which are called sutures. When this scheduled link-up fails to occur, a cleft palate is the result. Combined orthodontic and surgical treatment for patients with this defect begins nowadays quite early, in the hospital, and makes it possible for children with cleft palates to lead nearly normal lives. One thoughtful dentist, Dr. Bien, has speculated that it was precisely because such services were not available to him that Demosthenes made frequent trips to the sea shore. He was assembling a suitable collection of smooth stones to fill up (obturate is the technical term) the gap in the roof of his mouth he could close in no other way.

The mandible starts and finishes as one bone. It can't be victimized by clefts but very rarely parts of it fail to form. Neither does it make calcified junction with any other bone. Instead, it meets the skull, ball and socket style, just near the ears. Thus, at death, when the too, too solid flesh melts, thaws and resolves itself into a dew, the mandible becomes detachable. Until then you can feel the meeting (articulation) of the condyles, which are bony knobs atop the vertical part of the mandible (also called the ascending ramus), with the skull by placing your fingers next to your ear lobes and opening your mouth. It was a mandible, of course, that Samson used to slay one thousand men. Some of our late night entertainers can get the same results, also with the jaw bone of an ass, simply by talking us to death.

Picture the twenty baby teeth as being divided in half by being assigned ten apiece to each maxilla and these halves being divided equally again, into quadrants, by an imaginary center line passing from the tip of the nose to the center of the chin. With this floor plan in mind we can identify the teeth. (See figure 7.) The first in each of these quadrants,

Dental Data

next to the center line, is called the central incisor. Next to it, or immediately lateral, is the lateral incisor. All four mandibular incisors are slim and approximately equal in size. The maxillary centrals are larger than their neighbors, the graceful laterals. Moving down the line we come to tooth number three, the canine or cuspid (alias eye tooth in the maxilla and stomach tooth in the mandible.) We have suggested that teeth served in the evolutionary scenario for fighting as well as eating. Originally the canine teeth assumed a large share of that bellicose role. (Who can forget those exciting grammar school sessions devoted to prehistoric man that always featured dramatic views of a sabre-toothed tiger? They just don't make canines the way they used to.) Cuspids are shaped for piercing and tearing, incisors for shearing and scissoring (incising, to be exact.) The last two baby teeth are molars. Their task is grinding. Cows and horses and other animals that subsist entirely on grassy plants have only molars, which are kept busy because crushing up enough hay to nourish a cow is a full time job. All of the first or primary or baby or milk or deciduous (because they fall out, like the leaves of a deciduous tree) teeth usually erupt by the time the child is two years old. This schedule is widely and wildly variable. Sometimes an infant is born with a tooth already in place, which can give a mother who has planned on breast feeding something to think about, while another child may not get his first tooth until he's more than a year old. In neither case has the baby got anything to worry about, although the mother of the precocious child might. Generally speaking, the schedule of primary tooth eruption goes like this:

Central incisors	5 to 8 months
Lateral incisors	7 to 10 months
First molars	12 to 16 months

Cuspids .... 14 to 16 months
Second molars .... 20 to 32 months

Baby teeth practically never come in crooked. But occasionally the upper deciduous teeth may stick out. This condition will often be associated with a finger-sucking habit. It's best to ignore both the protrusion and the habit, as we have seen, until some permanent teeth begin to appear. Rarely, the lower primary teeth may protrude. Sometimes it's advisable to treat this Class III condition immediately. It's worth a visit to the orthodontist to find out. But in most cases treatment should be postponed until the eruption of at least a few permanent teeth.

What about those permanent teeth? We have already corrected Aristotle's alleged computation, putting the accurate count at 32. All of them will be considerably yellower than their deciduous predecessors, a state of affairs that dismays many people so much that they try vainly to restore the supposed milkiness. No whitener yet devised can have any success.

The eight permanent teeth in each quadrant, counting from front to rear, with their estimated times of arrival are:

Tooth		*Nickname*
Central Incisors	6 to 8 years	
Lateral Incisors	7 to 9 years	
Cuspids	9 to 12 years......	Canine, Eye Tooth
First Bicuspids	10 to 12 years	
Second Bicuspids	10 to 12 years	
First Molars	6 to 7 years......	Six Year Molars
Second Molars	11 to 13 years......	Twelve Year Molars
Third Molars	17 to 21 years......	Wisdom Teeth

Dental Data

The incisors and canines all replace their temporary counterparts which they resemble except in size and color. In addition to being yellower they are larger. That's why it's a good thing when spaces appear between the anterior deciduous teeth of a five or six year old child. This favorable development occurs during the final growth spurt for the front part of the jaws. If it doesn't the erupting permanent teeth are almost sure to be crowded. Two final comments about eruption scheduling: 1) lower teeth generally emerge before upper teeth, and 2) an indication that Begg may have been right with his attritional theory of occlusion is that when systematic extractions have been carried out the third molars generally appear much sooner than expected. It looks as though teeth that are allowed to drift forward either because of real or simulated (extraction) erosion leave enough room for the wisdom teeth to erupt on an earlier, possibly more natural, time-table, at 15 years or even before.

The last baby teeth to be lost are the temporary molars which may hang on until the child is 12 or 13. Under them, forming slowly for years have been the first and second bicuspids. They take their place in the arch when their predecessors have departed unless, of course, they have been selected for extraction by the orthodontist.

The next tooth in line is the six year molar, the first of the non-succedaneous teeth. It does not succeed anything. Because of this absence of a forerunner it often slips into the mouth unnoticed. Meanwhile, two more molars per quadrant are peacefully forming deep within the maxillae. Just at puberty, when great events are taking place elsewhere, the twelve year molars will make their appearance. Much later, at approximately the age when their possessor has been allowed to vote, the wisdom teeth will struggle into place. If anterior teeth, particularly in the lower jaw, which had, until then, been prim and orderly, seem to respond by buckling up, many patients and some dentists are quick to put the blame on the third molars. *Post hoc, ergo propter hoc.* There is no real evidence to prove a cause and effect relationship between the two events but prudent orthodontists may suggest removal of third molars in cases of corrected crowding where no other teeth had been extracted. On the other hand, sometimes wisdom teeth become impacted—prevented from erupting because they are wedged up against the teeth in front of them—even though bicuspids had previously been removed as an aid to treatment. If there is room for them, such misguided third molars can be surgically tipped back into place and allowed to emerge unhindered.

This rather complicated eruption plan does not always unfold without a hitch. At times it may appear that the child is sprouting a double row of teeth. This could be transient and no cause for alarm. Some balky baby teeth may just be making a delayed exit. But a more serious log jam may be forming, requiring a visit to the dentist.

Sometimes a large and unattractive space develops between the upper central incisors. This too may pass away. The laterals and then the cuspids tend to erupt diagonally, toward the midline, and as they emerge will seem to nudge the centrals together. But if the space is too large —it's called a diastema—or if the tissue between the centrals—it's called the frenum—is too resistant, dental help may be required. Perhaps the frenum should be removed or possibly the teeth should be brought together mechanically. Your orthodontist or dentist can tell you whether to wait or to seek treatment.

Without commenting on the timetable of their arrival, Cervantes once said that, "Every tooth in a man's head is more valuable than a diamond." Just what does this dental jewel of matchless price consist of? (See figure 8.) It has a crown, which is open for inspection whenever the lips are

Dental Data

parted, and a root which is buried in the gums and jaw bones. The crown is the part that gets cavities, that chews, whose orderly clean cut appearance wins rave notices when teeth are straight, and whose unhappy jumbles send patients to orthodontists when teeth are irregular. In other words, the crown is the part that gets all the credit when things go right and all the blame when they don't. But the buried portion, like the hidden bulk of an iceberg, may turn out to be crucial. For one thing, it is vital to orthodontic treatment.

Before examining the root in greater detail, we should take brief notice of the gums. This soft red membrane cloaks the bones of the jaw in the same way skin covers other parts of the body. But it is much more richly endowed with blood vessels than the skin which is a lucky thing for the dentist. Any cut he makes, planned or unplanned, is likely to heal quickly and without incident. Even so, the gums need care and exercise just as other organs and tissues do. The same rough diet that Begg speculated was responsible for attritional occlusion also gave the gums the daily work out they needed to keep their rosy glow of good health. Today, in addition to everything else that's wrong with them, our highly refined foods don't retain enough strength to give the gums any exercise at all. So stimulation must be provided by good brushing or proper use of dental floss, perhaps supplemented with irrigation with a pulsating water spray device. When appliances have been placed in the mouth it becomes more important than ever that teeth—and braces—be kept clean and gums be given plenty of exercise. Unfortunately, the design of many appliances makes it difficult if not impossible for dental floss to be used. So patients remove accumulations of plaque by brushing thoroughly, every surface of every tooth, at least once a day. This plaque is a thin, sticky film whose presence in the mouth is now felt to be the cause of decay and gum diseases.

Unfortunately many children, and some adults, are discouraged from massaging their gums because the neglected gingiva bleeds or hurts or both when touched. They proceed to cut down on their already inadequate schedule of brushing. Then not only do the gums continue to deteriorate but food and plaque also accumulate on the part of the tooth near the gum line. In time the area of the tooth under all this debris begins to rot. This process which is troublesome enough at any period can be disastrous if the chain reaction begins during orthodontic treatment. Then the vicious circle closes in more quickly than ever. Orthodontic progress may be seriously compromised, delayed, or even brought to a jarring halt.

The gums not only lie like a protective blanket over the jaw bones but a continuation of them also serves as a kind of hammock in which the teeth are suspended and by means of which are attached to the jaws. Teeth are not nailed into bone but are gently tied to it by countless threads of this gingival extension, the periodontal ligament. So if infection, caused by poor home care or anything else, attacks that outer layer of gum it will eventually spread to the periodontal ligament and then through it to the bone. This disease, when mild is called gingivitis and when serious periodontitis, causes the bony support for the teeth to weaken. Periodontitis, or pyrrohea as it is sometimes labelled, is the greatest single cause of loss of teeth in this country. Certainly no orthodontist wants to look into the mouth of a young patient and see what Groucho Marx claims to have observed behind the molars of a famous magician. The celebrated escape artist, the story goes, had secreted some of his props in his mouth. Grinning broadly, he asked a member of the audience, who turned out to be Groucho, what he saw.

"Pyorrhea," Groucho replied.

Whether enjoying good health or suffering from periodontitis, the periodontal ligament sends some fibers from bone to tooth; others connect one tooth with another. The outside layer of the root is the cementum. This material is almost identical with the bone that lies across the ligament. Almost, but not quite. Both have a capacity to resorb or break down. But while the ability of bone to repair itself is great, that of cementum is limited. Fortunately for the science of orthodontics, cementum is somewhat more resistant to resorptive forces than bone. Thus when force is applied to a tooth, the pressure is transmitted through the periodontal ligament to bone. Bone resorbs first (usually) and into this vacuum, so abhorred by Nature, the tooth will drift. On the tension side, where the tooth had been, specialized bone building cells get to work to lay down new bone. This alternation of resorption and deposit is the basic orthodontic process. After over 50 years of fairly intense research, no one has been able to prove conclusively whether it works best—whether a tooth can be propelled most effectively—with heavy, intermittent force or with light, continuous pressure or with some other combination. From time to time some fairly exciting piece of evidence, or just a bit of well phrased speculation, will trigger a wave of enthusiasm for a new appliance "philosophy." In the late 1950's, for example, Raymond Begg of Australia, Angle's brilliant pupil began to advocate a method that served as a therapeutic counterpart to his attritional theory of occlusion. He referred to it as a "light differential force" technique, claiming that by properly applying minimal pressures he could move anterior teeth backward speedily without disturbing the position of posterior teeth (This is just what's needed in the common protrusion: front teeth must be pulled into the mouth without dragging the back teeth forward.) There is no doubt the Begg technique works and works well. But so do some other methods that use much different levels of force and apply them in quite different ways. It may eventually turn out that there is no one best way to move teeth for all people or even all the teeth of just one person. Different patients and different situations may require individualized systems of force application.

But no matter what system is chosen, pressure must be directed against the crown of the tooth, which is covered by enamel, the hardest substance in the body. Readers who nourish hopes of physical immortality, apart from spiritual immortality, which is a topic beyond the scope of this modest text, would be well advised to pin their hopes on enamel. Because of the durability of enamel, teeth can survive their highly mortal possessors by hundreds of thousands even millions of years thus providing posterity with relatively imperishable anthropological evidence.

What the onslaught of century after century fails to accomplish, a tiny residue of pizza, chocolate, and cookies can achieve in a few months—destruction of enamel. Children, and adults, too, for that matter, who don't keep their mouths scrupulously clean are liable to get cavities. And braces, which can trap extra food particles, just make matters worse. Keeping the teeth clean, with a brush or with dental floss, is essential in preserving the health of teeth as well as gums. Good, daily home care is more important during orthodontic treatment than at any other time.[1]

In order to protect Cervantes' jewel, the enamel encrusted tooth, three parties must do their jobs: 1) First, the orthodontist should make appliances that fit well, that offer no nooks and crannies in which food can adhere to start the decay process. Then, the orthodontist, or an assistant, can check regularly to see that the braces remain intact and well sealed, 2) Second, during check-up visits,

Dental Data

family dentists can satisfy themselves that all appliances, like Caesar's wife, are beyond reproach and that any uncovered teeth are free of decay, and 3) The patient himself should maintain a daily program of cleaning and inspection to see that no part of his appliance has loosened. With this kind of shared vigilance, orthodontic devices that might otherwise pose a threat to the health of the dentition can actually, by sealing teeth off from oral fluids, preserve them from harm. Thus a potential aggressor can be persuaded to turn not only the other cheek, but also the other lip, tongue, and tonsils, too. (See figure 13)

If, in spite of all these combined precautions, dental decay gains a foothold and passes through the enamel, it will reach a somewhat softer but still mineralized tissue, dentin. There are no pain fibers in enamel, so any assault on this first line of defense may slip by unnoticed. When decay reaches dentin it may or may not announce itself by causing a toothache. Up until this point, any damage can be repaired with a regular filling. But if decay manages to invade the final dental citadel, the nerve, or pulp, as dentists call it, special measures must be taken. This pulp, the soft tissue vital center of every tooth, is filled with nerves and blood vessels. Because it is entirely surrounded —and imprisoned—by calcified and rigid dentin, it has no room to manoeuver; swelling is not a defense mechanism available to it. The pulp has only one response to insult more serious than a momentary blushing—it dies. A blow from a bat, or a fist, or a ball, or the edge of a swimming pool can do it. Or infection from any source can cause the pulp to succumb. But it is unlikely that any orthodontic manipulation could be sufficiently traumatic to stifle the vitality of even the most delicate tooth.

Should the worst occur and the nerve die, all is not lost. The pulp can be removed and replaced with what is called a root canal filling. Teeth treated in this way lose most of their vital functions but retain some capacity to interact with their surroundings thanks to the periodontal ligament. Teeth with successful root canal fillings can survive as long as any other and may even wind up some day submitting to the bemused inspection of an anthropologist of the distant future.

TABLE OF ILLUSTRATIONS

Figure I—Class I Occlusion

Figure II—Class I Malocclusion

Figure III—Class II Malocclusion

Figure IV—Class III Malocclusion

Figure V—Cephalometric X-Rays

Figure VI—The Brain Cases of Ape Man, Early Man, Modern Man

    The Jaw Bones of Modern Man and Primitive Man

Figure VII—Human Dentition

Figure VIII—The Human Tooth

Figure IX—The Orthodontic Appliance—Active Phase

Figure X—The Orthodontic Appliance—Extra Oral

Figure XI—The Hawley Retainer

Figure XII—The Orthodontic Appliance—The Positioner

Figure XIII—Surgical Resection

Photographic Illustrations:
    Varieties of Malocclusion—1-7
    McGraw and Tutin's "Belle"

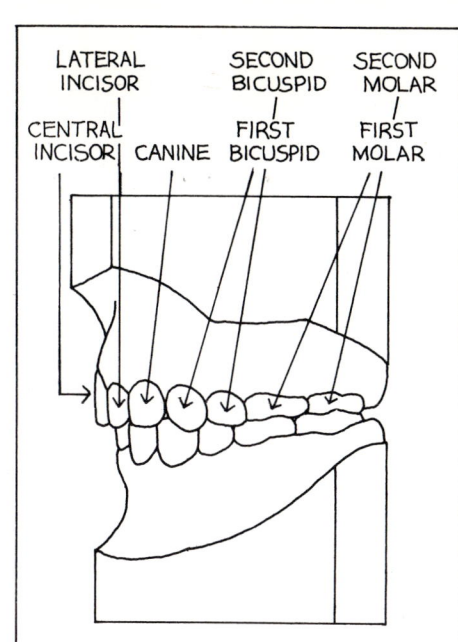

FIGURE I.
CLASS I OCCLUSION.
An "ideal" bite.

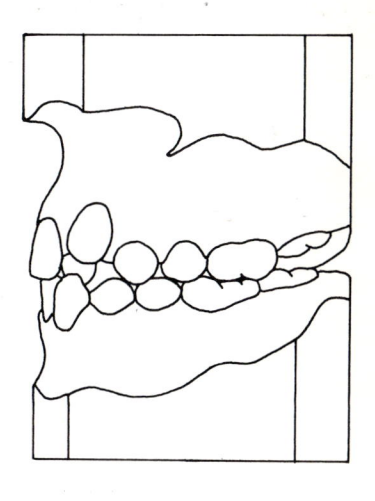

Labels: CENTRAL INCISOR, LATERAL INCISOR, CANINE, FIRST BICUSPID, SECOND BICUSPID, FIRST MOLAR, SECOND MOLAR

FIGURE II.
CLASS I MALOCCLUSION.

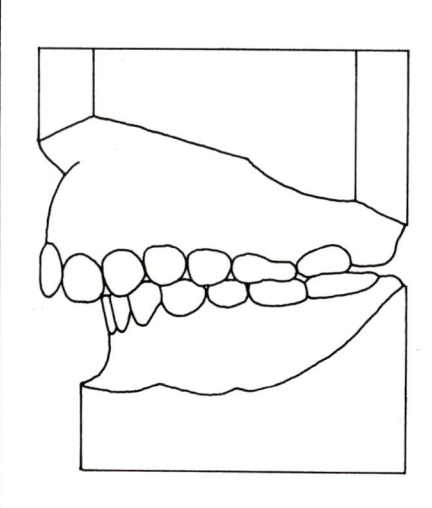

FIGURE III.
CLASS II MALOCCLUSION.
Upper Teeth Sticking Out.

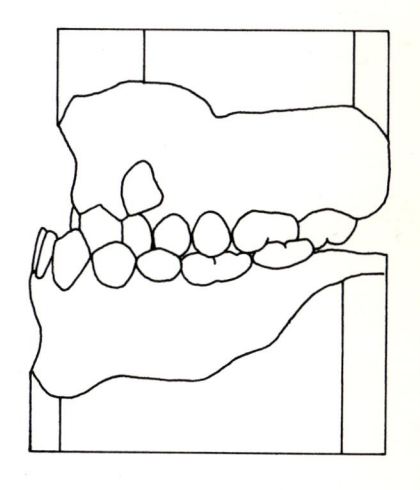

FIGURE IV.
CLASS III MALOCCLUSION.
Lower Teeth Too Prominent.

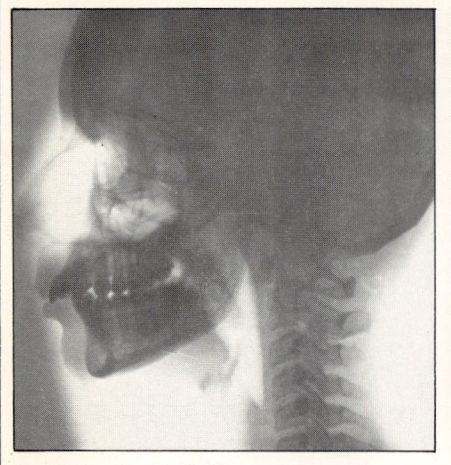

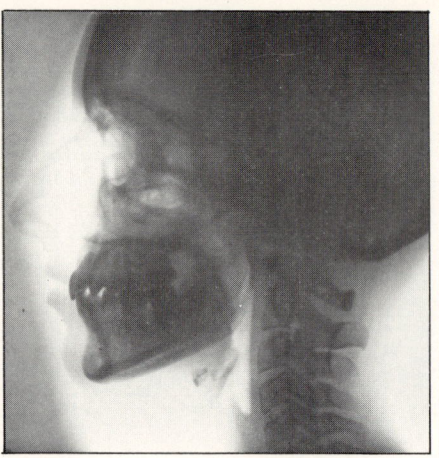

Before — After

FIGURE V. These cephalometric (head measuring) X-Rays allow the orthodondist to survey the problem and, after treatment, to determine just what he has done.

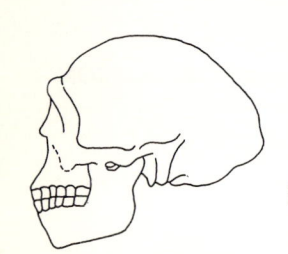

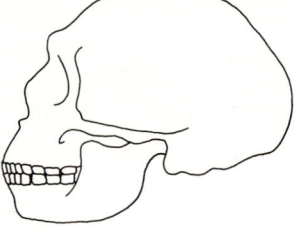

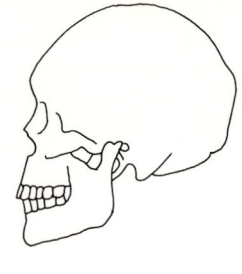

A. Ape Man   B. Early Man   C. Modern Man

FIGURE VI. The brain case advances as the dentition retreats in the progression from ape-like ancestor to modern man. This increases our capacity to think but leads to increasing problems in chewing our daily bread.

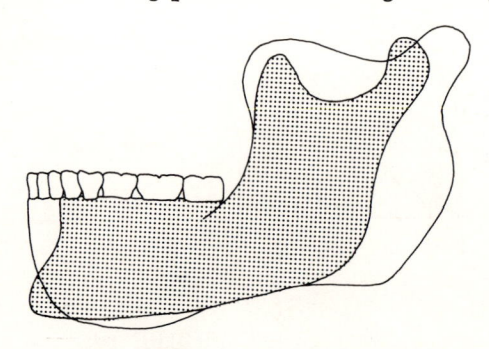

D. A relatively delicate modern mandible superimposed on the jaw-bone of a primitive man.

HALF FRONT VIEW

▦ Baby Teeth
☐ Permanent Teeth

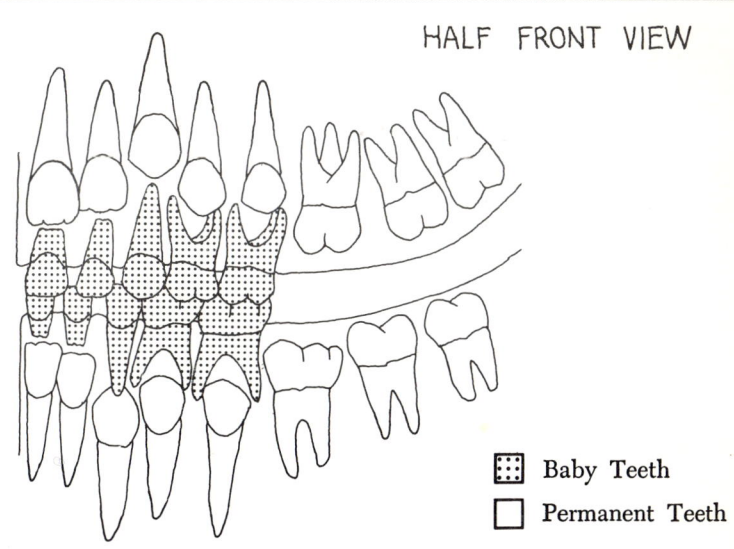

FIGURE VII. THE HUMAN DENTITION.
The human dentition consists of four quadrants of five baby teeth which will be followed by four quadrants of eight permanent teeth, making a total of twenty deciduous teeth and thirty-two permanent teeth.

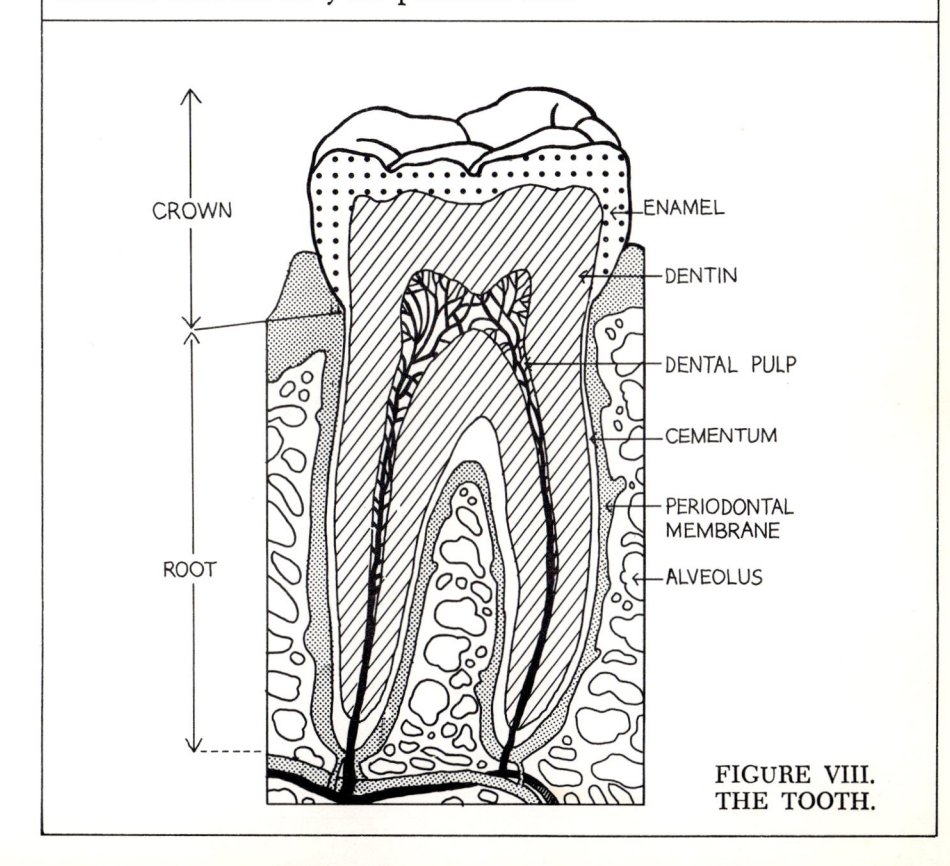

CROWN

ROOT

ENAMEL
DENTIN
DENTAL PULP
CEMENTUM
PERIODONTAL MEMBRANE
ALVEOLUS

FIGURE VIII.
THE TOOTH.

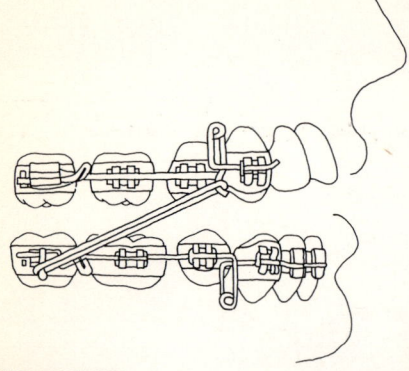

FIGURE IX.
THE ORTHODONTIC APPLIANCE.
Active phase.

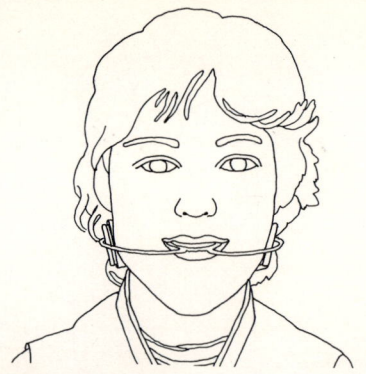

FIGURE X.
THE ORTHODONTIC APPLIANCE.
(Extra oral) Night Brace.

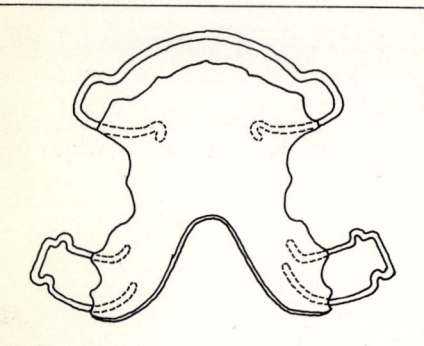

FIGURE XI.
THE HAWLEY RETAINER.
A removable device widely used to prevent straightened teeth from back-sliding.

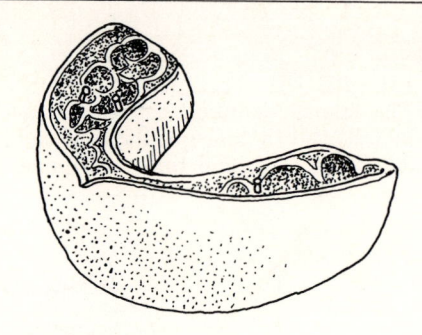

FIGURE XII.
A POSITIONER.
A rubber mouthpiece molded on an idealized set of the patient's teeth. It is an alternate kind of retainer.

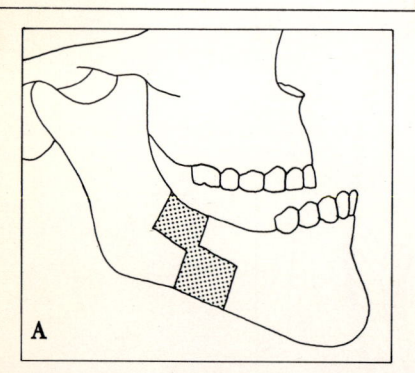

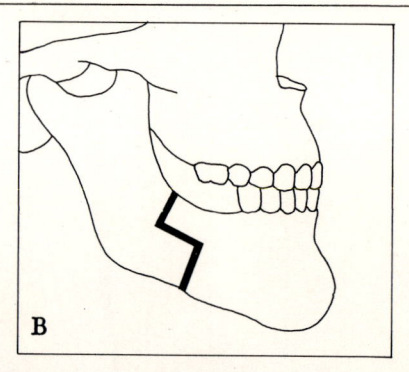

FIGURE XIII. SURGICAL RESECTION.
This severely protruding jaw can be corrected surgically. In one type of operation the dotted area (A) is removed and the anterior portion of the lower jaw is set back into correct occlusion (B).

THREE VARIETIES OF MALOCCLUSION

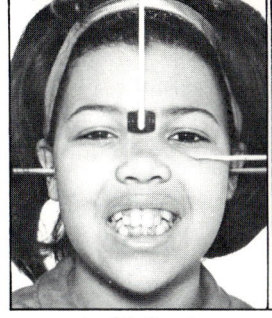

CLASS I MALOCCLUSION. CROWDING
Four teeth removed, one in each quadrant.

A (Before) A 1 (After)

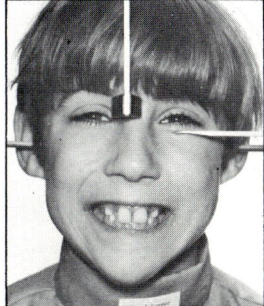

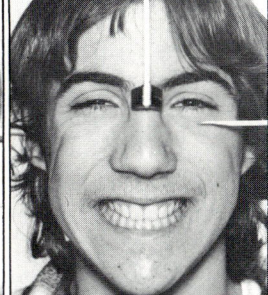

CLASS I MALOCCLUSION. AN ANTERIOR CROSSBITE.
The upper lateral incisors were locked behind the lower anterior teeth.

B (Before) B 1 (After)

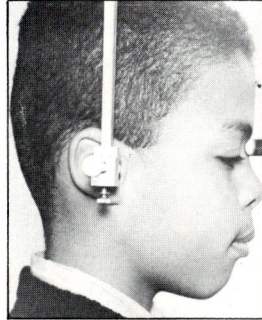

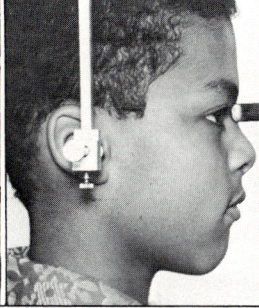

CLASS I MALOCCLUSION.
In this bi-maxillary protrusion, the removal of four bicuspid teeth provided room for the retraction of the incisors.

C (Before) C 1 (After)

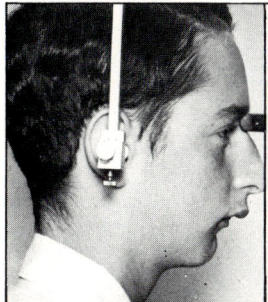

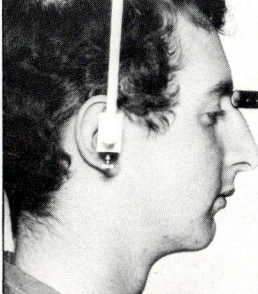

CLASS II. MALOCCLUSION.
A successful orthodontic result was due, in no small part, to the exceptional cooperation of the patient in wearing night brace and rubber bands.

D (Before) D 1 (After)

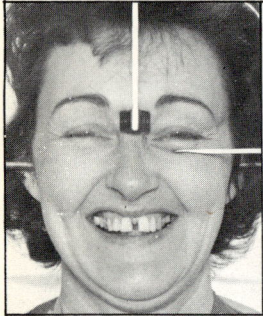

E (Before) 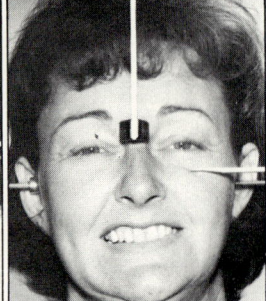　　E 1 (After)

CLASS II MALOCCLUSION. An example of adult orthodontics. A space between the central incisors was corrected.

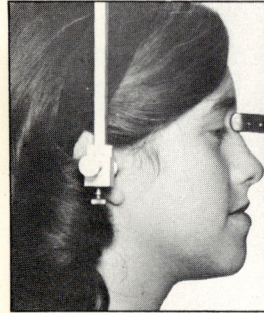

F (Before) 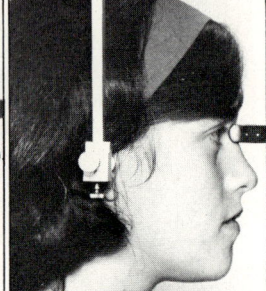　　F 1 (After)

CLASS III MALOCCLUSION. Protrusion of the lower teeth is much less common than other types of malocclusion.

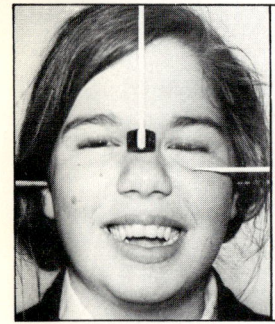

G (Before) 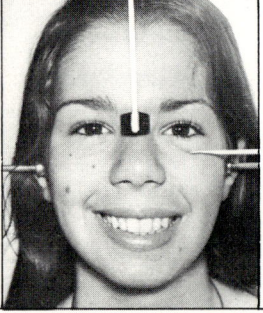　　G 1 (After)

AN OPEN BITE. This patient was so pleased with the correction of her open bite that she promptly lost thirty-five pounds.

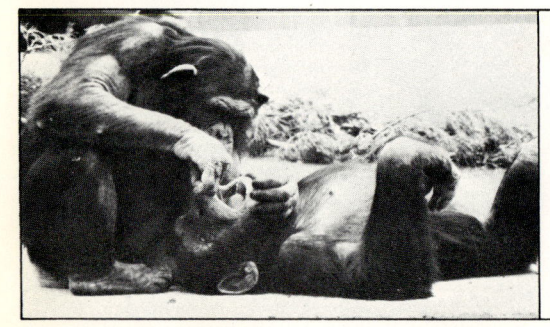

BELLE. H One of the chimpanzees observed by McGraw and Tutin. Chimpanzees take better care of their teeth than some orthodontic patients.

All photographs taken by Dr. Jay Weiss, except for the picture of Belle.

Chapter Ten

THE "RIGHT" AGE TO SEE AN ORTHODONTIST

> I have bought
> Golden opinions from all sorts of people.
>
> Shakespeare, *Macbeth,* I, vii.

In trying to decide when to seek an orthodontic opinion many people have as much trouble as Shakespeare's Hamlet who hesitated so much in making up his mind that "his native hue of resolution was sicklied o'er with the pale cast of thought." Of course, if either the family or school dentist has suggested a visit, this problem of timing swiftly disappears and the native hue of resolution has a chance to perk up a bit. But suppose a parent notices his child's teeth swerving abruptly from what he considers to be a normal and disciplined standard. They may be sticking out too far, they may be crowded, or, like certain arid stretches of the Far West, be too generously provided with wide open spaces. Can a worried parent take matters into his own hands and make the orthodontic appointment himself? Why not? He has nothing to lose but his pains. Even if the doctor puts the child off and advises a return visit in a year or so, the initial examination may provide useful insight about the direction and pattern development is taking. Such knowledge can be helpful later in planning an appropriate individualized treatment plan.

If each case must be judged on its individual requirements, what are some of the general considerations that orthodontists evaluate in deciding when to begin therapy? Here is a brief assessment of the chief categories:

Cross Bite—Most orthodontists agree that all cross bites, anterior or posterior, even in the deciduous dentition, ought to be dealt with soon after they are discovered on the theory that they constitute an interference with the orderly unfolding of development. As deciduous teeth are moved from their faulty cross bite positions to their proper places, the permanent teeth, hidden above them in their bony crypts, follow right along.

Lower Protrusions—If these consist of nothing more than a few teeth biting incorrectly they can be regarded as cross bites and, accordingly, corrected promptly. But if the lower teeth are stuck in front of the upper teeth because the mandible is growing too exuberantly, the orthodontist will have to choose between treating early, attempting to guide apparently unfavorable growth along more desirable lines, or adopting a policy of skillful neglect and waiting until he can be sure orthodontic treatment makes any sense. For a very few of these mandibular prognathisms wind up with such large lower jaws that only surgery can right the wrong committed by a negligent fate. By distinguishing one category from another it may be possible to uncover the exremely rare cases for which early treatment would simply be a wasteful expenditure of effort that would only have to be repeated at a later date. Generally speaking, lower protrusions caused by a poor relationship between teeth can can be handled with braces; those that reflect a more serious lack of harmony between bones, or skeletal parts, may eventually require an operation.

Upper Protrusions—Very few orthodontists like to treat these in the deciduous dentition when only baby teeth are present but some do want to get started in the mixed dentition when deciduous and permanent teeth coexist amicably. Again, they take the view that whenever a road block clogs the path of normal development it's wise to eliminate it so that Nature can resume its steady flow in the right direction. Often treatment can begin as soon as the six year molars and permanent anterior teeth have fully erupted, at about the age of nine, particularly if lower teeth are straight and well positioned. But if there is a likelihood that teeth will have to be removed, treatment can't reasonably commence until the candidates for extraction have reached a place where they can be hustled off the stage without too much gory and damaging surgery. This may mean braces can't be used until the patient is 12 or 13 years old. Even when extractions aren't contemplated many orthodontists prefer to await the arrival of the adolescent growth spurt, a period when rapid maturation carries the bones of the lower face downward and forward away from the cranium. Different parts of the body grow at different rates. A child of eight has completed most of his cranial growth; the lower face doesn't achieve adult dimensions until about age 13 in girls and 15 or later in boys. By timing their treatment to coincide with growth, orthodontists try to encourage forward movement of the mandible and restrain the maxilla, which is already protruding, from coming any further forward. The combined efforts of an orthodontist and properly guided forces of maturation can produce startling changes in facial appearance. (See fig. 14)

Other reasons for postponing therapy include the desire of some practitioners to include 12 year molars in their treatment strategy and the unsuitability of some techniques for management of malocclusions in the mixed dentition. Thus, to some extent, at least, orthodontists are limited by the capabilities of the appliance they habitually employ.

Other experts, notably Charles Tweed,[1] have argued that it's foolish to stand, or sit, idly by while teeth stray into positions of maximum disadvantage. Why not intervene as early as possible, they reason, since "there is a tide in the affairs" of teeth "which taken at the flood, leads on to fortune . . . we must take the current when it serves."

Tweed and others have shown excellent results with such early treatment. (See fig. 15) In addition to the mechanical benefits that accrue from minimizing the distance that teeth must be moved, there are also some compelling psychological arguments for treating children before they reach puberty. These will be discussed in chapter 12.

Spacing—This is one condition which, like wine and cheese, can improve with age. All other malocclusions of permanent teeth are almost sure to remain relatively unchanged unless treated orthodontically. So the answer to many a parent's inquiry, "Won't my child outgrow this condition?" is usually short. "No."

But since the upper canines have a tendency to erupt toward the mid-line it is generally prudent to wait until chances of self-correction have been exhausted before starting to close spaces between teeth. If the thick tissue between the two central incisors—the frenum—needs to be removed, sometimes it's best to have this done before treatment and sometimes after. You'll have to rely on the judgment of your orthodontist or oral surgeon, who will actually perform the minor operation, to decide what timing is best in your case.

Crowding—This condition is easy to recognize. It frequently stimulates an anxious parent to hurtle into the nearest orthodontic office demanding to know how serious a problem that "double row of teeth" is going to be. Sometimes the alarm is false. A baby tooth or two may thoughtlessly have overstayed the allotted time even as replacements were already slipping into place. When the reluctant baby teeth depart the problem will disappear along with them.

Serial Extraction—Other crowding conditions refuse to go away. Oddly enough, the most severe of these shortages of space can be the easiest to deal with. Some seven year old children seem to have only about half the room that will be needed to accommodate the emerging incisor teeth. Studies have shown that growth in the front part of the mouth is virtually completed by this time. So Mother Nature can't be expected to help out. One solution, which was introduced roughly twenty years ago, calls for the removal of selected baby teeth at proper intervals to allow each successive permanent tooth to erupt unmolested into its proper place in the dental arch. Of course, this is a temporary, steal from Peter to pay Paul, solution. No room is created. As with a game of musical chairs, the odd tooth in the quadrant is the one eventually to be left in the cold. In a well-executed program of serial extraction, that is exactly the game plan; the odd tooth out is extracted as soon as it appears in the mouth, sometimes before. This move is timed to allow all the other permanent teeth to come in as close to target as possible without having to be moved mechanically. In Class I cases, where neither an upper nor a lower protrusion complicates things, this serial extraction approach can be quite successful. But always serial extraction must be employed with care. It can cause more problems than it solves. And even when it works, it must frequently be supplemented by mechanical orthodontic treatment to tidy up the remaining ragged edges.

In cases where crowding is not severe, serial extraction does not provide a ready answer. There is no way to extract a fraction of a tooth from each quadrant. Yet this is all the room that may be needed. Some compromise may be called for: stripping, modest expansion, selection of teeth other than first bicuspids for extraction. And always, of course, the orthodontist should be sure that the anticipated benefits of his ministrations will clearly outweigh the difficulties of his treatment.

Space Maintenance — From time to time, owing to unchecked decay or other calamities, a baby tooth may be called to its reward years in advance of schedule. Suppose the dearly departed is a first or second deciduous molar. Will the teeth behind it tend to press forward with all the eagerness of a $2 gambler who has finally backed a long shot winner after a series of disastrous losses? You bet! Is it always necessary to prevent this from happening? Not necessarily. In cases where there is no crowding, where there are no problems with the "bite," yes, the space should be maintained for the eventual eruption of the permanent tooth that is waiting in the wings. But in the kind of crowding for which a program of serial extraction, as outlined above, may be indicated, the construction of a space holding device would be a futile enterprise.

Chapter Eleven

MOLAR MECHANICS: WHAT ALL THOSE LITTLE GADGETS ARE FOR AND HOW THEY WORK

> But it does move!
> Galileo Galilei, *from* Abbe Irahilh, *Querelles litteraires,* 1761, III, p. 49.

The first duty of any branch of the healing arts is to prevent trouble from happening in the first place, to nip disorders in the bud if they do get started, and only as a last resort, to apply extensive therapeutic measures to cure full blown maladies. At the present state of orthodontic knowledge, preventive techniques, like serial extraction, remain limited in number and effectiveness. So, in order to cure the large number of malocclusions that still slip through barriers erected by current, relatively primitive public health schemes it remains necessary to direct some sort of force against Tooth A to move it from point X to point Z pausing as briefly and effortlessly as possible at intermediate point Y.

Why can't appliances that deliver the required power be inconspicuous and why can't they be detachable for Junior Proms or Big Games? Well, sometimes they can. When teeth are slightly spaced or just a trifle irregular, a removable device equipped with a few wires or springs may be all that is needed to tip teeth into position. Sometimes an uncomplicated, clear colored plastic splint can be cemented over a few teeth to cope with a routine cross bite. It will do the job in a matter of weeks or months.

And, as will be seen in chapter 13, a whole new world of plastic see-through braces is beginning to take shape.

For the present, however, their cosmetic benefits are not always readily available.

Some elaborate removable appliances—one of the most sophisticated is named after its originator, Dr. Crozat—have been designed to avoid the grim necessity of being too obvious. They are used principally for expansion, generally by dentists who believe that expansion will cure most orthodontic ills, and are not mechanically capable of accomplishing anything more than the tipping of teeth. When that is all that is needed, they can serve a useful role. But there are times when teeth must figuratively be picked up by the scruff of the neck (teeth actually have a neck—at the junction between the crown and the root) and moved bodily in any of four directions—up, down, backwards or forwards—or in some artful combination of these major possibilities. When such exquisite control is called for there is, as yet, no way to avoid cementing attachments to all or most of the teeth. With cemented, or fixed appliances, it is possible to apply force in a steady, reliable way at two points on tooth surface thus developing bodily movement or translation in space of the tooth. Only in this way can anterior teeth be pushed into the bone, or intruded, to correct a closed bite or extruded to eliminate an open bite. Only with fixed appliances can spaces left by extracted teeth be closed properly; without them crowns could be moved together but roots would be left at least as far apart as they were to begin with. If the kind of procumbent teeth that give the well known television personality, Bugs Bunny, his characteristic appearance were simply tipped toward Mr. Bunny's throat, they would wind up leaning backwards, looking "dished in." With fixed appliances performers like Mr. Bunny, whose faces are their fortune, can have the roots of their teeth moved almost as readily as the crowns. This capability of uprighting tipped teeth allows today's orthodontist to rescue precariously leaning teeth from outlandish attitudes that can be unhealthy, unstable, and unattractive.

Angle devised a number of appliance systems, the last of which, called the Edgewise technique, was introduced in the middle of 1920's. It remains perhaps the most widely used, in a variety of guises, of the fixed appliance methods. Other fixed techniques include Begg's system, also in great vogue, the Johnson twin arch, the Universal technique, and the labio-lingual system which relies largely on tipping forces. The removable systems can be divided into two groups: those that apply force directly to individual teeth like the Crozat and those that endeavor to transmit muscle power, of lips or cheeks, to groups of teeth through the intermediary of a large plastic device called an activator or a mono-bloc. These latter are popular in Europe but not generally employed in this country.

Despite this bewildering variety of mechanical approaches, beginning orthodontic patients anywhere in the United States are likely to share a series of puzzling experiences that will follow each other in an order something like this. After having submitted to the record-taking procedures described earlier and having learned what general plan has been adopted, they will presently find that little metal objects are being placed between many of their teeth. What's up? Or in? And why? Those pieces of metal are not the long awaited braces but are separators which, like John the Baptist crying in the wilderness, herald a greater arrival soon to come. In a few days the teeth are gently forced apart so that bands can be fitted and then cemented. During their short stay the separators are a source of vague irritation, usually nothing more.

The orthodontic bands themselves serve as a means of securing attachments to teeth and are contoured strips of thin metal cylinders that fit tightly around a tooth like ski pants over the legs of Jean-Claude Killy. The attachments, which are welded to the bands, are designed to receive arch wires which will do the actual moving, guiding, or holding of teeth. Many of the bands also carry buttons or cleats welded to the lingual side. They are used as hooks for attaching elastic pressure or as an auxillary place to bind teeth together. The terminal tooth in this arrangement, a molar in each of the four quadrants, carries a tube; the other teeth are equipped with brackets. (See figure 9.)

In Angle's day all of the band construction had to be done laboriously by hand and all attachments had to be soldered in place, one by one. He used precious metal and needed to squeeze a magnifying monocle into one eye in order to be sure he hadn't inadvertently sealed off some important opening or carelessly severed some joint no man should ever have put asunder. Now most bands and attachments come prefabricated like a ready-to-wear copy of a Paris gown. They usually fit much better than either an Angle original or a Gimbels copy. And if he does have to hook on some attachment, the modern orthodontist or his assistant can weld the parts together because the material used is stainless steel. The welding process is much simpler than soldering and requires no eye-piece which is one reason Ernie Hixon commented that orthodontists were getting out of the jewelry business.[1]

Bands may be constructed directly in the mouth or made indirectly on a model. The process of fitting and cementing is tedious but doesn't hurt. Because of the time required and the care needed to seduce attachments into the most effective of all possible positions, orthodontists usually insist that patients be excused from school for the two to five long initial visits that such an exacting encounter demands. Later, adjustments can be made during short after school appointments with occasional major overhauls requiring additional absences from the classroom.

As many as 24 bands are placed in each case which is why the Angle, Begg, and similar methods are known as multi-banded techniques. Learning to live with these fixed appliances can be difficult. Patients must pass through a variable period of adjustment before lips, cheeks, and tongue get used to the sudden invasion of troops of brackets, tubes, buttons, and cleats. (The attachments, in turn, are humming, "I've grown accustomed to your face" in slightly tinny tones.) At this time, and throughout treatment, irritating rough edges can be smoothed over with a bit of wax or clay or even chewing gum until the orthodontist can be reached for emergency help.

If teeth are to be extracted, this may be the moment for it. The orthodontist, who does neither fillings nor extractions, will refer his patient back to the family dentist or to an oral surgeon to have teeth pulled. If the procedure is complicated or if the patient requests general anaesthesia, it is probably best to visit a specialist for the extractions. But when there is no objection to local anaesthesia, which is administered with a needle or to the removal of four teeth in two visits, two at a time, most general dentists are perfectly willing and fully competent to do the job.

Ten days to two weeks later active treatment will begin. The initial arch wires, one for each jaw, can now be eased through the molar tubes and secured to the brackets on the other teeth. Often the first wires will be light and highly resilient, especially if the arch form is irregular. By means of their built-in elastic force they will begin restoring order not only among teeth that have strayed from the *horizontal* limits of propriety but also even off obstinate canines or incisors that had insisted on settling themselves at different *vertical* levels. By applying the right amount of gentle force, orthodontists can even tease into the chorus line impacted teeth that had strayed so far out of place that they had to be uncovered by an oral surgeon. The trick is to pit one force against another—for every action there is an equal and opposite reaction, Isaac Newton used to say as he bit thoughtfully on an apple. While the flexible wire pulls the tooth that is too close to the tongue it pushes with identical fervor on the tooth that is bumping into the lip. In instances where no such reciprocal exchanges can be arranged, the plot thickens.

Many situations, alas, are not suited to simple give and take displacement or up and down interaction. When all the teeth of one jaw, or even the jaw itself, need to be pushed back toward the tongue, as in a Class II or III malocclusion, additional sources of power must be sought. Archimedes explained long ago that if he only had "where to stand" and a sufficiently long lever he could move the world. Orthodontists have similar but much more modest specifications. They, too, need a place to stand. They call it anchorage. Also required is a means of applying the force.

If, for example, upper teeth stick out, as in the case of Mr. Bugs Bunny, lower teeth can be joined together with some kind of appliance so as to form an anchorage unit. Elastics can be worn from the posterior, or distal part of this unit to hooks placed in the anterior part of a similar appliance on the upper jaw. The elastic action of the rubber bands will pull the protruding upper teeth back into the mouth. Since, as Newton pointed out, for every action there is an equal and opposite reaction, the lower teeth will tend to come forward just as much as the maxillary teeth will be inclined to go back. Sometimes this is a good thing. Sometimes it isn't. The lower teeth may *need* to come forward but often they already have enough anterior inclination. In such cases the orthodontist will either want to extract lower bicuspid teeth so that incisors can be up-righted and *then* enlist in the effort to supply a source of anchorage for retraction of protruding upper teeth, or it may be advisable to look for a place of anchorage somewhere else, outside the mouth.

This is where head gear or night braces or home braces come in. With such devices, whatever they are called, the elastic force is anchored on top of the head or in back of the neck and is applied either directly to the protruding anterior teeth or to molars on the theory that posterior teeth must be corrected first before incisors can be brought into line. (See figure 10.) In addition, timely pressure aimed against molars can modify directional growth of the jaws, slowing forward movement of the maxilla while encourag- the mandible to sail along unimpeded. In an Andy Gump kind of face where the chin is conspicuous by its absence this combination of events is highly desirable. Of course, the head and neck are just as subject to reciprocal rebound as lower teeth but they are too strong to show any adverse effects. They do move but their mass is so great in comparison to the protruding teeth against which they are pitted that the net effect on them is inconsequential. (The same thing happens when a ball is thrown to the ground. Both ball and earth react equally, but the volume of the earth is large enough to make its response infinitesimal while the ball can take some highly visible and occasionally crazy bounces.) Because Newton's laws have not yet been repealed, orthodontists always suspect that patients whose teeth move sluggishly or not at all simply aren't wearing elastics or night brace as prescribed.

After records have been taken and appliances assembled and installed, subsequent appointments are spaced at one to six week intervals depending on current progress and degree of cooperation.[2] A checkup visit may consist of nothing more than a verification of the integrity of wires and bands or it may be the occasion for a change in arch wires or some other substantial mechanical revision. Because progress is variable, it is seldom possible to know in advance whether an appointment will take five minutes or two hours. Parents and friends who accompany orthodontic patients would be well advised to make the trip armed with a suitable diversion—a good book, a topic worthy of prolonged meditation, or an extensive shopping list.

While all this is going on orthodontists want their patients to continue seeing their family dentists on a regular basis. But they usually find it impossible, except under unusual circumstances, to remove appliances every six months. Taking off 20 or 24 bands and putting them back on again two times a year would become an ordeal for patient and orthodontist alike. So, to insure dental health during orthodontic treatment, the following precautions are taken. First dentist and orthodontist check carefully to see that all cavities have been filled before bands are cemented. The orthodontist then makes the best fitting appliances he can because a tightly sealed band actually protects a tooth while a poorly adapted band can cause decay. If a space develops between band and crown, food will pack into it and lead to etching of the enamel surface. Orthodontists and their assistants are on the lookout for such breakdowns on each visit. The patient's responsibility in this joint venture is to keep his teeth clean—for some young people a heavy burden, indeed—and even to inspect his own bands from time to time to see if any have loosened. And, finally, the family dentist contributes his third party observation to be sure all is well.

As the teeth move closer and closer toward home base the orthodontist can insert increasingly rigid wires, each one more nearly approximating an ideal arch form than its predecessor. After each manipulation teeth are likely to feel tender for anywhere from a few hours to as long as a week. If there is no sensitivity, possibly nothing is happening. But if *too* much pain persists, the orthodontist may wish to adjust the adjustment by loosening a wire or two.

Sometimes patients will complain that their teeth are getting too loose. Some amount of looseness is normal and necessary—without it no orthodontic movement would be possible. As was seen in Chapter 9, the teeth are suspended in the periodontal ligament, a kind of a hammock, and even without the pressure of braces would occasionally be prey to a vague feeling of flexibility. Of course, too much looseness could be a danger signal. The dentist can judge when that wobbly sensation is appropriate and when it isn't.

And so, slowly, imperceptibly, in answer to the orthodontic siren call, teeth slide into line. How long will it all take? That depends on the difficulty of the case and the extent to which the patient heeds the orthodontic commandments: Thou shalt wear thy rubber bands and thy headgear. Thou shalt keep thy teeth and braces clean. Thou shalt not covet bubble gum nor anything else that is tough and sticky neither shalt thou covet thy neighbor's caramel or salt water taffy. (Beyond avoiding chewy substances that can distort delicate wires and springs there are really no dietary restrictions for the orthodontic client. However, many patients may voluntarily choose to select a menu stressing soft foods and liquids after a strenuous adjustment. Biting into anything hard may become temporarily awkward.) The simplest of cases that unravel without a hitch may be completed in something over a year. A realistic time-table for the average problem will be about two years. And, of course, when the malocclusion is severe or cooperation is scant, or some combination of the two slows down progress, therapy will take even longer.

A rocky road, perhaps, but one worth traveling for many young people. What about the adult population? Can a grown up be a suitable candidate for orthodontic treatment? Yes. So long as his gums and supporting bone are judged to be healthy enough to withstand the strains of appliance manipulations. Any malocclusion that can be corrected for a child can be managed almost as well for a healthy adult. Whatever added impetus that might have been supplied by adolescent growth will, of course, be absent in the treatment of grown ups. In addition, while children grow accustomed fairly quickly to the slings and arrows of outrageous appliances, adults find the breaking in period considerably more taxing. Root moving is also more difficult with adults than it is with young people. Because of these limiting factors, it is often prudent to set standards for adults at a somewhat lower level than for children, but generally speaking, treatment proceeds for one group in the same way it does for the other.

In addition to the general kinds of malocclusion that are found among adults, certain special situations arise. Sometimes a dentist is prevented from constructing a suitable replacement for a missing tooth because its mates have strayed out of line or tipped into awkward postures. Orthodontic ministrations, like bull dozers leveling the approaches to the Hudson River, can prepare the way for an adequate bridge. Because it is the ultimate in fixed appliances—a dental bridge is planned to last a life time—it should maintain whatever corrective work the orthodontist may have done in anticipation of its placement.

This kind of built-in guarantee would be much appreciated by all orthodontists winding up treatment but is rarely available. Orthodontists regret this because at times they must stand grimly by and watch their noblest efforts slowly buckle up and drift back toward the configuration of the original malocclusion. The name of the problem is relapse. Like the poor it has always been with us and

Molar Mechanics

though heaven and earth might pass away relapse will doubtless abide.

How come? For one thing, the original malocclusion had a certain stability or it wouldn't have survived. Entrenched muscle patterns that have helped to create and sustain it may persist after treatment ends. They will urge teeth to slip back into their former evil ways. The fibers of the periodontal membranes that encircle and cradle teeth will join in this anti-social enterprise for they are elastic and are possessed of a kind of molecular memory. While they may appear to submit meekly to orthodontic pressures, they will eagerly reassert themselves at the first opportunity. One worker has suggested that this type of collapse can be forestalled by trimming over stretched fibers that are poised to spring back, dragging teeth along with them, as soon as restraint of appliances has been released. This approach has never become popular.

In his last published article Hixon described his attempts to plan treatment so that no stabilization procedure, mechanical or surgical, would be required.[3] Following Hixon's reasoning, an orthodontist would never force teeth into spaces normally occupied by lips or cheeks. In short, he wouldn't expand and he would extract teeth when necessary. But even if they subscribe, in principle, to this Hixon Doctrine, most orthodontists are reluctant abruptly to abandon straightened teeth without some kind of guardian to watch over them.

One of the first and still the most widely used device designed to keep potentially unruly teeth in line is the Hawley retainer, named after the Washington, D. C. orthodontist who introduced it in 1919. (See figure 11.) Made originally of vulcanite, a rubber-like material, and now of plastic, it is a removable plate that fits over the palate or behind the lower teeth and carries a wire that presses around the anterior teeth and prevents them from moving. It can be worn continuously or just at night depending on the needs of the case. A variety of similar plastic retaining devices has been introduced, some with, some without, wire auxiliaries. No one is quite sure how long they should be used. Many a cautious orthodontist will simply urge his patient to keep on wearing the retainer at night until it dies a dignified death of old age; the retainer, not the patient, although in extreme situations an exasperated orthodontist might settle for either one.

Like Sarah Bernhardt who kept on coming back for one more farewell appearance, the return of lower incisor crowding seems to be a perennial repeat performer. To protect against it, some orthodontists use fixed retainers. They either salvage lower cuspid bands from the original appliance or make new ones. A rigid wire is soldered between the two bands in such a way that it tightly and accurately engages the lower anterior teeth. The device, called a lingual arch, is cemented in place. As long as it is worn the lower incisors have no more chance of eluding restraint than a mental patient has of escaping from a strait jacket. But a lingual arch suffers from the same defect that plagues any other retainer, or strait jacket: once the patient is freed from confinement he is likely to slip right back into his old patterns.

In the 1940's a dynamic approach was tried. At the conclusion of treatment, or even before it, an ideal model of the patient's teeth was constructed. It was made by improving an actual model of the patient's dentition. Any teeth whose position left something to be desired were cut off the model and reset in a better position. Then, over this idealized model, a rubber mouthpiece was molded. The patient, whose teeth occupied stations in life almost, but not quite, on a par with those of the corrected model would bite into the mouthpiece for four hours a day, while he studied, or watched television, or simply sat around reflecting on why he had no time to take out the garbage. Sometimes this device, called a positioner, coaxed teeth into the most attractive possible arrangement. But sometimes, in spite of it, a certain amount of relapse occurred anyway. (See figure 12.)

Third molars, as we have seen, have frequently been cast in the shifty role of villain in this drama. Although there is no hard evidence to prove their guilt, extraction of these teeth may avoid trouble in some cases particularly when there is little or no room for them.

Another solution proposed for the recurring problem of lower incisor relapse has been inter-proximal stripping. It is still too early to tell how much of an answer this relatively new technique will provide for one of orthodontics' most perplexing questions.

Still another method of coping with relapse was popularized by the Begg technique. Instead of merely turning a rotated tooth to a corrected position, Begg suggested that orthodontists keep right on spinning it considerably beyond the desired angulation. Then, when the inevitable occurred, the treated tooth would "relapse" to the spot the orthodontist wanted it to inhabit in the first place. This basic principle of over-treatment can, in fact, be applied to all aspects of orthodontic therapy. A maxillary protrusion can be treated *beyond* the ideal upper incisor to lower incisor relationship, an open bite can be closed down a little excessively, and a closed bite can be transformed into one that is slightly open. "This overmovement," Begg says in his text, "causes the forces that move teeth toward their pretreatment positions to be dissipated by the time the teeth move back to the positions they should finally occupy."[4] Unfortunately, he neglects to explain just why this should be so.

Does the distressing tendency of teeth to slip backward mean that all attempts to persuade a stubborn malocclusion to accept permanent reform are predestined to fail? Not at all. A healthy respect for the diabolic inclination of teeth to backslide can enable prudent practitioners and patients to deal with it. By selecting a sensible treatment plan that will not defy established muscular behavior or overtax usable space and by executing an appropriate program of retention, the orthodontic team may not be able to eliminate slippage entirely but it can usually contain it within acceptable limits.

Some readers may be forgiven if they lose interest in the narrative and interrupt to inquire anxiously, "Yes, yes, very interesting. But how much is it all going to cost?"

In 1972, a university clinic in the East was charging $850 for standard two year treatment. Private fees, of course, are higher. They vary from perhaps $900 to $2000. Most orthodontists prefer to set a fixed fee, adjusting it only in exceptional circumstances no matter how long or how short the actual treatment period turns out to be. It is customary to ask for a substantial appliance fee which, after decoding, means down payment, with the balance payable over a two year period in monthly, or any other convenient, installments. If retainers are lost or broken through carelessness, most orthodontists charge between $40 and $60 for replacements.

Chapter Twelve

BUT SOMETIMES THOSE GADGETS DON'T WORK AT ALL. HOW COME?

>Just like a tree that's standing by the water, we shall not be moved.
>
>Old Union Song

Peter Blos, the author of *On Adolescence* and *The Adolescent Personality*, is generally regarded as the country's leading psychoanalytic authority on the problems teenagers face in growing up. When asked what impact he thought issues of self-esteem would have on the course of orthodontic care he reflected on those of his patients who were reclining concurrently on both psychoanalytic and orthodontic couches. "Of course, some of the adolescents I had in treatment also received orthodontic treatment," he wrote in a kind and perceptive letter. "There was less of a body image involvement or disturbance, rather more an active rejection of body function interference ('keep this stuff out of my mouth . . .'). This seems to be due to the fact that orthodontic treatment is, more often than not [undertaken on] the parents' initiative and consists of their 'corrective interference' with the child's body and its 'defectiveness.' It is rather, therefore, the parents' body image ideal of their child that complicates orthodontic treatment." [1]

However true this interesting bit of speculation may be, it is certain that *something* interferes with the orderly transformation of crooked teeth into responsible members of the dental community. Dr. Jerome Weiss, a thoughtful New Jersey orthodontist, commented recently, "Mechanical advances of recent years have made it technically possible for us to achieve a good correction of most malocclusions.

But some patients just don't respond the way we think they should. And these always seem to be the children who cooperate very little or not at all." [2]

Good cooperation from clients is crucial to orthodontic therapy in several ways. Unless teeth and appliances are kept clean, decalcification and decay of teeth may result no matter how well constructed the appliances may be. Gums may also become sore and inflamed which may not only be a problem in itself but will also slow down tooth movement. Raw and swollen gingiva will resist the advance of orthodontic forces as stubbornly as the Greek guard at Thermopylae. And if a client does not wear elastics or head gear at least part of the allotted time there can be no correction of a protrusion.

Every orthodontist is painfully aware that very few of his patients do everything he asks them to do and that some of his patients do almost nothing he asks them to do. And the situation may actually be much worse than he thinks. In fascinating unpublished studies conducted at Loyola Dental School by Drs. Campisi, Cavanaugh, and Gannon,[3, 4] a group of patients who "had told their orthodontist that they always wore their elastics and headgear the required time" were confronted with a lie detector. These hardened grammar school desperadoes promptly broke down and "admitted being unfaithful." Then, when they were actually "tested by the polygraph they were found even less faithful" than they had just confessed to being. In fact, the boys' measured truthfulness score for elastic wearing was a stunning 26.6%. Girls earned slightly better marks. When quizzed about the length of time they submitted to the constraint of a head gear, the boys earned honesty grades of 53.3%, not enough, perhaps to put them in a class with George Washington or a high grade Eagle scout, but still an improvement on the elastic level. Dr. Campisi guessed that "the fact that the headgear was obviously visible" made lying about it difficult and unconvincing.

Why should patients find it more convenient to stretch the truth than their rubber bands? Well, elastics hurt, at least when they are put on for the first time. It's easier to "forget" to wear them than to put up with mild discomfort. They can be a nuisance, too. All of this ought to be perfectly obvious. But orthodontists seem singularly unwilling to discuss this aspect of their craft. The present writer once submitted an article entitled "Some Psychological Aspects of Dental Pain" to a European orthodontic society. The piece, which eventually appeared in *The New York State Dental Journal*,[5] was rejected on the ground that the subject was not relevant to the practice of orthodontics. Indeed, pain, and its management, is a topic that gets little attention in the journals of any orthodontic society. Occasionally, however, a back-handed reference to this phantom issue slips by the informal defenses. In a brief communication explaining the difficulties that would attend any attempt to remove all bands for every routine dental checkup, Saul Kaye argued that to do so would be "tantamount to re-doing the orthodontic set-up every 6 months. Aside from the tremendous loss of time involved, it is a constant repetition of a painful treatment phase for the patient."[6] Apparently, the average orthodontist ordinarily sketches his *own* self image along lines that stress slick but gentle healing and ignores any rough stuff.

But he can quickly adjust the picture if he has to for the sake of argument. His procedures, he contends, never hurt the first time. It is only when he is asked to repeat them that he is willing to discuss the possibility that they might become traumatic.

Actually a concerned orthodontist can manage to execute all his manoevers without causing any sustained physical discomfort during office visits. By being patient, by listening, by explaining, he can clear up the mystery about what he is going to do. This is usually enough to comfort even the most timid patient. Troubles usually don't start until the client takes himself and his new appliances back home. Even before real tooth movement begins, some of the braces, as we have seen, can cause irritation to tender lips, cheeks, or tongue. Then, of course, when pressure is applied a certain variable sensitivity may develop several hours later and persist for anywhere from half a day to almost a week. But for most people the chief complaint about braces is the same one that keeps divorce courts working over time. It isn't so much physical abuse, it's mental anguish that leads to all the suffering.

In the first place, children are concerned about what one of the Loyola investigators referred to as "social impediments." In his study Gannon found that "prospective patients ... possessed a great desire for orthodontic treatment." But later he discovered that "the majority of patients" actually undergoing it seemed "to hold negative attitudes." Out of twenty children interviewed in midstream, nine replied to the question, "would they be willing to do it all over again?" with a flat "NO," six were undecided, and five were willing.[7]

What causes this sharp decline from an apparent high level of desire to something much lower when treatment moved from the planning stage into high gear? Probably many things. As Blos pointed out, the body image needs being served may be parental or dental and have little to do with the patient himself. For another thing, the patient's views on the matter may be ambivalent. He would certainly like to reap all the gaudy financial, social, and sexual advantages that Madison Avenue assures us are bestowed on the owner of a dazzling smile, but all that is tomorrow. Today, appliances are annoying. It takes a certain amount of maturity to be able to postpone gratification as required by the Reality Principle instead of cherishing the immediate delights of bubble gum and caramel as advocated by the Pleasure Principle. To compensate for the short supply of maturity found in the patient population, sophisticated parents and orthodontists might learn to offer prompt reinforcement for desired behavior as suggested by Skinner's Operant Conditioning.

For another thing, no matter what their surface significance may be, the appliances may constitute a latent threat. D. Montandon of Geneva put the thing quite neatly when he observed, "Quel que soit l'âge auquel on opère une malformation congenitale de la face, cette intervention représente une aggression traumatique, aussi bien du point de vue physiologique que psychologique." Succinct. To the point. (No matter at what age one operates on a congenital malformation of the face, this intervention represents a traumatic aggression, as much from the physiologic as from the psychologic point of view.) Montandon continues that, nevertheless, "this psychological trauma can't be compared with what the patient would have to endure throughout his life if no correction were undertaken." [8]

In psychoanalytic terms, the insertion of appliances may be construed as a sexual attack. One moderately disturbed female patient tearfully refused to wear a head gear because she said, "It will get stuck." Neither would she permit the use of any instrument she perceived to be "penetrating." Similarly, adolescent boys, according to Selma Fraiberg writing in *Adolescents, Psychoanalytic Approach to Problems and Therapy*, have "a morbid dread of homosexual contact with an adult male." [9] This kind of thing could make it difficult for a patient to concentrate on his rubber bands.

According to Judith Essig, a behavioral scientist studying the sociology of dentistry at Columbia University, adolescents may also be concerned about possible limitations imposed by appliances on what they can eat and what they can do.[10] These fears, as the poet says, are really "foolish fancies." All orthodontists do insist, for good reason, that their patients eliminate bubble gum, caramel, taffy, and other tough and sticky confections that can make the braces look as though they'd just been paid an unexpected visit by Attilla the Hun. Most other foods, eaten carefully and sensibly, remain on the approved list. It's true that some adjustments make chewing of anything difficult, but such sensitivity is only temporary.

As far as talking is concerned, braces, except for the short lived annoyance of some removable devices, don't interfere with it a bit. They may even help by giving a bashful teenager something to talk about.

There isn't any reason orthodontic patients have to cut down on physical activities, either. Properly protected with mouthguards, boys can continue to participate in even the most vigorous contact sports like football. Wrestling seems to produce more damage to appliances than any other endeavor, but repairs can be made when needed. Boys should not be discouraged from taking part in sports if they wear braces or from wearing braces if they take part in sports.

For many years orthodontists worried that pressure from musical instruments could have a harmful effect on tooth position. Very little suspicion ever fell on the piano or the drums but it was feared wind instruments with inside the mouth embouchures, like the clarinet, would contribute to an upper protrusion. The trumpet, on the other hand, could help to *cure* a Class II malocclusion. The flute was considered to be neutral. Nowadays, orthodontists are much more relaxed than they used to be about wind instruments and simply advise their patients to be careful to adopt a good embouchure which will not only help them to play well but will also protect their incisors from unfavorable forces. But will braces make it difficult for young musicians to play? Not usually. Beginning and intermediate players won't be affected at all. But top level musicians may find orthodontic appliances a real hindrance. Any concert grade performer ought to consider this possibility carefully before he decides to begin orthodontic treatment.

Adolescent girls, Essig continues, will be less likely to worry about limitations on their athletic activities than on their burgeoning sexuality.[11] A suburban orthodontist wondered aloud recently, in the presence of his 15 year old daughter, if teenagers were really concerned about the comic strip possibility of braces locking as an aftermath of a passionate embrace. "Well, they don't need to worry about it, Daddy," she said. "I can assure them it doesn't happen." This, of course, is the real nature of the "social impediment" the Loyola research team euphemistically described.[12] Many former patients can attest to the fact that the impediment is more imaginary than real. On that magic day when appliances are finally removed, the glowing escapee returns to family and friends beaming widely, anticipating scenes of wild celebration and unconfined joy. To his chagrin, *nobody notices*, not even the parents who have paid the bill and listened to anguished complaints for the preceding two years.

Another large group of patients may have something else to worry about. Being sentenced to suffer the removal of four teeth may be a severe emotional blow to some children. As Schoenberg and Carr pointed out in *Loss and Grief: Psychological Management in Medical Practice,* there is a great "likelihood that the patient will mourn any change or loss of a body part." Teeth especially have great significance. They are said to be the unconscious symbols of virility or femininity. Patients should be encouraged "to discuss the anticipated loss as well as . . . feelings following the change." [13] In his work on the effects of "fear-arousing communications" Janis has stressed the importance of providing patients with plenty of advance information about what is going to happen to them. The "work of worry" can then be utilized to diminish apprehension. When it finally arrives, an event that has been thoroughly "rehearsed mentally" will be less anxiety-provoking than one that comes as a relative surprise.[14]

For these, and doubtless additional, reasons, orthodontists are going to be confronted with recalcitrant subjects. Unfortunately, they may not be ideally suited to deal with these emotional problems. Reviewing the literature for the American Association of Dental Schools, Crowder reported in 1966 that the dental profession "attracts a rather constricted type of individual and one who is rather compulsive, materialistically oriented, culturally restricted and tradition-bound." Crass citizens such as these, archetypal of what the Freudians call an anal character, would seem less than ideally suited for gentle coaxing of reluctant patients into desirable patterns of behavior.[15]

But the effort ought to be made. It is one way an orthodontist, together with parents, can improve the cooperation of unwilling patients. From the beginning, children should be made to feel that they are active participants, that they are working *with* the orthodontist not being worked *on*. They should participate in making decisions so that they will not fall victim to the tyranny of authoritarian control.

Some orthodontists have despaired of ever obtaining enough cooperation to make their treatment proceed smoothly. In their book, *Becoming a Dentist*, Sherlock and Morris have described such types as "a common personality ... in dentistry: cautious, orderly, persistent, conservative, and interested in the applied rather than the theoretical." [16] Instead of trying to understand what makes patients resist orthodontic correction, they assume total control by tying appliances in place. Explaining how this is done, one lecturer recently entitled a short presentation, "24 Hour Per Day Headgear, I like it." [17] In this system patients wear their headgear to school and everywhere else, as well as to bed, because they cannot take it off. Advocates of this method argue that permanent headgear is no more handicapping to a patient than a cast on a broken limb. And it certainly speeds up treatment. It is also possible to use a system of coil springs instead of elastics in the mouth and tie them in place. No studies have as yet been published on how patients feel about such tactics. And, of course, it may be difficult, indeed, to uncover the impact, on the deepest psychic levels, of permanent headgear and coil spring elastic forces.

There is another way to capture that elusive ingredient, cooperation, without actually lassoing it and chaining it down. Orthodontists simply need to select patients who *want* to cooperate. And they should try to avoid those clients who are predisposed to engage in exasperating power struggles with adults. According to psychoanalytic theory the early school age child is going through a stage, the latency period, during which he would like to please adults, not overpower them. That is what makes him ready to channel his abundant energies into the task of mastering readin', 'ritin', and 'rithmetic and that is what makes him a potentially excellent patient. By the time this paragon of orthodontic virtue reaches puberty he is plunged again into a bewildering effort to assert his independence and he finds himself assaulted by incessant instinctual demands boiling up from the deepest levels of his unconscious mind. That is why he so frequently neglects to clean up his room and finds it absolutely impossible to wear his rubber bands. From the point of view of the orthodontist, he is a vicious specimen indeed. Yet this embittered revolutionary is the very character designated by many orthodontic systems as the ideal candidate for correction of dental irregularities.

But in many cases it is not only possible but even preferable, from a mechanical point of view, to begin treatment with nine and ten year old children. No less an authority than Charles Tweed, it will be recalled, became an advocate of early treatment. By beginning orthodontic care promptly, he argued, he could encourage teeth to erupt close to the location he had mapped out for them instead of allowing them to wander into the worst possible positions from which they would later have to be forcibly ejected. Then, to his surprise, Tweed discovered that instead of being management problems, these younger clients were actually better patients than the older children he had been accustomed to treating. Gannon, at Loyola, discovered the same thing. "The older age group (twelve years eight months to eighteen years) was less willing," he said, "to tolerate the social impediments involved during treatment than the younger age group (ten years two months to twelve years eight months.)" [18]

With Dr. Harold M. Eiser I have been testing the hypothesis that the emotional storms of pubescence make it a time of life ill suited to the exacting demands of orthodontic treatment. In addition to their Oedipal struggles with parents and parental figures, adolescents are also confined by the constraints of their group codes. Blos describes a "defense . . . prevalent in American youth" which he calls *uniformism*. "It is a group phenomenon which protects the individual within the group against anxiety, from any quarter. The boy or girl who does not fit into the particular uniformism which is established by a given group is usually considered a threat; as such, he is avoided, ridiculed, ostracised, or condescendingly tolerated." [19] If the group standards do not include the wearing of head gear, or braces, or rubber bands, the luckless adolescent orthodontic patient is going to be caught in a tug of war between peer pressure and dental requirements. Eiser and I are finding that while there is little difference between age categories in the wearing of rubber bands, orthodontists do indeed perceive their adolescent patients to be considerably less reliable in the use of head gear and removable appliances than younger patients. It is easy to see which team usually wins the tugs of war.

It is not so easy for many people, whether they are patients, orthodontists, parents, or merely bystanders, to realize that orthodontic therapy consists of something more than just a confrontation between two forces: the orthodontic appliances and the resistance of the patient's teeth. Often the delaying tactics of the patient himself are stronger, more determined, and more durable than even the most stubborn resistance displayed by an entrenched malocclusion.

Chapter Thirteen
NOW YOU SEE THEM, NOW YOU DON'T: SOME POSSIBILITIES FOR THE FUTURE

> Every valley shall be exalted and every mountain and hill shall be made low: and the crooked shall be made straight, and the rough places plain.
>
> Isaiah, XL, 4.

When Lincoln Steffens returned from a visit to the Soviet Union in 1919, he proclaimed that he had "been over into the future, and it works."[1] Observers of the orthodontic scene, and this includes virtually anybody who glances into the mouth of a passing suburban teenager, may occasionally have the same eerie sensation. The inconspicuous plastic brackets that will someday remove orthodontic appliances from the category of "social impediment" are already making a leisurely and bashful appearance in high school hallways and soda fountains or wherever it is that adolescents hang out nowadays. But, while they are present in modestly increasing numbers, these modern plastic braces aren't much noticed in teen age haunts. They pass by unperceived not so much because there are still relatively few of them in circulation or because there is so much smoke (from cigarettes and other things) in teen age haunts to reduce visibility. The reason is simple. Plastic brackets are transparent, at least to begin with. When they age, they tend to pick up stain. But, as technology improves, they may become the answer to the sensitive patient's complaint, "Why do my braces have to be so noticeable?".

It was Bernard Baruch to whom Steffens made his startling if not entirely accurate pronouncement. Baruch received the information with an understandable absence of enthusiasm. Many orthodontists feel the same way about the new-fangled plastic gadgets.

According to George Newman, a practicing orthodontist and also an adjunct research professor at the Newark College of Engineering, the skeptics had better take a long hard look at the new devices, and soon. Newman, who was the first to introduce an epoxy bonding system in the early 1960's, is convinced that, "Within the next two to five years some type of plastic attachment will have gained wide acceptance by the public and the profession alike, at least for the upper anterior teeth." As bigger companies grow interested in the marketing possibilities in orthodontics, Newman predicts that, "You're going to see one hell of a change." [2]

Traditional orthodontic bands have always been supporting players, a necessary evil. Orthodontists have known that as soon as someone devised an effective way of attaching brackets, tubes, and buttons directly to teeth, the days of the middleman, the orthodontic band, would be numbered. The search for an adhesive that would be strong enough to withstand chewing pressures, which can soar as high as 30,000 pounds per square inch, go right on working under water, like a deep sea diver, and at the same time be non-toxic, led Newman through a complicated maze of formulas for resins including acrylics, cellulose nitrates, polycarbonates, nylon, polysterenes, and vinyls. These were just the "more promising" thermoplastics. Newman also sampled the thermosetting group, including epoxies, polyesters, melamines, and allyl diglycol carbonate. Working with a team of engineers and chemists at the Newark College of Engineering, Newman first came up with an epoxy that performed nicely in the lab. But would it do just as well in some trusting child's mouth? Facing this kind of crucial question, medical investigators really have only one choice open to them. They try it on themselves. When Walter Reed was struggling to uncover the means of transmission of Yellow Fever there was no way to confirm his theories without experimenting on human beings. Reed seemingly proved his case in one of the great demonstrations in the history of preventive medicine but several of his colleagues sacrificed their lives in the process. Sigmund Freud, a codiscoverer of the anaesthetic properties of cocaine, had a happier experience. He sampled the stuff and loved it. "In my last depression," he wrote his fiancée, "I took coca again and a small dose lifted me to the heights in a wonderful fashion. I am just now collecting the literature for a song of praise to this magical substance." [3]

Newman's experience fell midway between those of Freud and the associates of Reed. It didn't kill him but he didn't exactly enjoy it, either. Here is how he recalls the episode: "We made the first bonded attachments by hand from clear cure acrylic, shaped them individually with dental instruments, and polished them. I bonded them onto my upper incisors with an epoxy adhesive. After the attachments had been on my teeth for two weeks they began to yellow and I tried to remove them with a dental pliers. I can recall standing before my bathroom mirror perspiring freely while the attachments refused to budge. My diet, subsequently, consisted of lamb chop bones, chicken bones, and spare ribs. I tried pressing the brackets with forks and spoons but, to no avail. I even chewed bubble gum. I was afraid I'd break off tooth enamel when I removed the attachments and then have to explain the missing tooth structure to colleagues and patients. This occurred in 1956 before there were any reports in the literature on bonded attachments. I finally gnawed on enough chicken bones to loosen the bonds and was able to snap the attachments off with my pliers. But I felt as though I was twisting my teeth out of their sockets." [4]

Manipulation of this material gave Newman other troubles. He developed a contact dermatitis, tried wearing rubber gloves, and then abandoned epoxies entirely. Next he shifted to an acrylic resin that satisfied most clinical requirements without giving patient or doctor a rash. But so far neither Newman nor anyone else has succeeded in formulating a bonding agent with the marvelous stickiness of that first, 1956 compound. He's still checking out new chemicals in the lab and just to be safe he keeps a large supply of chicken bones in his refrigerator at home.

The next big problem was to simplify the bonding procedure itself which was highly complex. Orthodontists who, as Hixon put it, had only recently been liberated from the tedium of the jewelry business were not going to be overjoyed about having to slip on an alchemist's robe and begin boiling up agents and reagents that might gum up their practices disastrously. Newman and other pioneers throughout the world have managed to eliminate much of the cumbersome preliminary work required for the bonding of an attachment that will stay put when needed and be removable with relative ease when its work has been finished. "Similar problems," Newman says, "are faced by various marine, oceanographic, aviation, and space industries. Somebody is bound to come up with improvements that will be just what we need, provided we can get FDA approval." While at present only plastic brackets can be made in appropriately clear tones Newman feels that eventually their more sturdy metal counterparts will be produced in tasteful enamel colorings and be capable of accepting a durable bond to tooth surface. When that day comes, almost certainly within the next decade, orthodontics may continue to be as uncomfortable as ever but it will be far less obtrusive than it is now.[5] The next move, of course, will be up to the 24-hour-a-day boys. Will they make head gear in the form of ear muffs?

And, of course, in order to camouflage the presence of braces really effectively, it will be necessary to use not only brackets that melt into the countryside but wires that will be able to do the same thing. Newman is certain that these, too, will arrive on the scene some time in the next decade. Then, the objective that he described in a 1964 article of creating an orthodontic system that would allow "oral hygiene [to] be improved and aesthetics to be enhanced" [6] will seem so close that the profession, aided by its special skills, will almost be able to taste it.

There are still other indications, some already appearing in scattered orthodontic waiting rooms throughout the country, of what the future holds in store. Some are old friends. For, as Sir Patrick Cullen remarked to the recently knighted Sir Colenso Ridgeon in Shaw's *The Doctor's Dilemma,* "Modern science is a wonderful thing. Look at your great discoveries! Look at all the great discoveries! Where are they leading to? Why, right back to my poor old father's ideas and discoveries . . . Don't misunderstand me, my boy. I'm not belittling your discovery. Most discoveries are made every fifteen years; and it's fully a hundred and fifty since yours was made last. That's something to be proud of . . ." [7]

The technique of rapid palatal expansion didn't have to wait quite so long to be found again in this country. It was first developed by the American Angell around 1860; was abandoned here some fifty years ago because Angle, Case, and others feared it was too dangerous a procedure; and finally reintroduced in the United States about 100 years after it first saw the light of day. Europeans, notably the German school, had never stopped relying on rapid expansion since it harmonized with their basic approach to orthodontics. This method, which so alarmed Angle and his followers that they relegated it to the dental dust bin, consists of rigidly attaching a jack screw between the left and right posterior teeth of the upper jaw. The screw is opened steadily, one or two turns a day. Very quickly, after several days, the two halves of the maxilla, which join in a mid-line suture, are actually separated. Then swiftly, they are pushed apart. Within two weeks an opening of up to 15 mm. (a half inch) can be created and, oddly enough, without pain.

By the time most people are about 17 years old, the two halves of the upper jaw have made a bony union and palate splitting is no longer possible, although in some cases the suture can stay open until well into the 50's. But for younger patients this expansion device directs its force against bony structures, not teeth. Thus it can properly be considered an orthopedic (bone moving) not just an orthodontic (tooth moving) appliance. Since the floor of the nose and the roof of the mouth are one and the same, this technique can also hold out promise of relief for patients with breathing difficulties. Because it spreads out the upper jaw more or less permanently—even with this orthopedic method a certain amount of relapse must be anticipated—it is particularly useful in cases where the upper arch is narrow and pinched in. It is also clearly indicated in Class III cases where there is often a marked insufficiency of the upper jaw. While most of the widening force spreads the maxilla laterally some of it tends to thrust anterior teeth forward. This is good in Class III cases but bad in Class II cases with narrow upper arches where the incisors are already protrusive. Advocates of the technique claim it reduces the need for extraction of teeth, others contend it plays a useful role when upper arches are narrow and expansion is clearly needed but that none of the basic criteria determining whether or not teeth should be removed is altered in any significant way.

But the enthusiasts do not rest their case there. They claim that the rapid expansion device is just the first of a whole host of true orthopedic appliances. In recent years these workers, some of whom tend to align themselves with the 24-hour-a-day school of thought, have claimed that by applying heavy, continuous force they could do more than just split the maxilla like Moses parting the waters of the Red Sea. With pounds of pressure, not the customary ounces, they contend they are moving many of the bones of the facial complex. They do it with chin caps and by stepping up the pressure of conventional head braces. Some of the ailments that are said to respond to these heroic measures include severe open bites and both maxillary and mandibular protrusions. Suggestive of the enthusiasm being generated by and among proponents of this approach is the title of one article published in 1970, *Palatal Expansion: just the beginning of dentofacial orthopedics.*[8] Skeptics, who included, not surprisingly, the late Ernie Hixon, insisted that while rapid expansion certainly moved bones it would remain the only truly orthopedic tool orthodontists were ever likely to use. Forces of large magnitude and duration could, of course, mold the facial skeleton, Hixon conceded to a friend one night in 1968 after a session of the French Orthodontic Society. This is clearly demonstrated by the Milwaukee brace which orthopedists use to treat weak backs. It encases most of the body in a cast for long periods. Because it also presses against the chin the Milwaukee brace has the unhappy side effect of compressing the mandible. No doubt either, Hixon admitted, that by means of ritual binding the Chinese were able to reshape women's feet to an extent not even dreamed of by Thom McCann shoes. Some African tribes have done equally impressive things with collar size by clever application of necklaces of a type that are not available in local jewelry stores. But such forces are too strong and must last too long for an orthodontist to consider using similar means, Hixon said. All that can be stated with assurance about the future of orthopedic treatment in orthodontics is that the issue remains very much in doubt.

European practitioners, for whom the impact of American theories has been blunted by the broad expanse of the Atlantic Ocean and two World Wars, do not tend to use such ponderous methods, except for rapid expansion which they perfected, but many of them claim they have been applying orthopedic forces for years, anyway. They do it, they say, with the activator which was developed by the Norwegian, Andresen, in the 1930's. He got the idea from Pierre Robin, a Frenchman whose original apparatus, introduced at the turn of the century, was known as the monobloc. Today there are many variants of the basic design, each with a different spring or screw built in, one for almost every province in Europe. All of them consist of a rather cumbersome one piece design which receives the lower teeth on its underside and accommodates the top teeth on its upper surface. Activators are made of acrylic (or sometimes a light metal like aluminum) and act to force poorly positioned lower jaws to bite in only one way, the preplanned "right" way. Gradually new reflex patterns are supposed to be developed so that in time the mandible will not only assume a reformed position but will also grow into a more favorable shape. The underlying theory resembles the one proposed to the 98 pound weaklings of America by Charles Atlas. By constant repetition the Atlas scheme of exercise transforms feckless flab into effective muscle. Similarly, the story goes, a retiring mandible can be guided, by *functioning* in a programmed way, into the desired size and outline. This is the *functional* basis of European style jaw orthopedics.

Not possible, American academic orthodontists have insisted. The size of the mandible is genetically predetermined and cannot be altered by man, appliance, or Presidential proclamation. So ingrained is this attitude that even Tom Graber, an enthusiastic advocate of dento-facial orthopedics, American version, argued in the third edition of his popular text (1972) that so-called functional devices are bulky, require a higher degree of cooperation than most children are likely to extend, take longer than fixed appliances and can't achieve as detailed a result, work only during periods of active growth, are actually more difficult to use than American methods, and, finally, "may produce permanent damage" because a "jiggling effect" is produced where "the appliance [shoves] the teeth one way and the functional forces [push] in the opposite direction." [9]

Egil P. Harvold, a Norwegian orthodontist-researcher, who studied under Andresen, makes far less extravagant claims for activators. Currently Professor and Chairman of the Department of Orofacial Anomalies at the University of California Dental School in San Francisco, Harvold practiced orthodontics in Oslo for 18 years. At the end of that time he reviewed his records and found he had used activators in 50% of his cases and that in roughly half of those, he had to finish treatment with a full-banded appliance. This means he judged activators to be fully effective for less than one fourth of all malocclusions. This is scarcely a high enough percentage, he adds, to make the device the public health panacea some advocates have claimed. In a course given at Fairleigh Dickinson University in May, 1974, Harvold said that he had never been able to grow bone with an activator and that he had never seen any evidence proving anyone else could do it. Instead, he said, activators work on a less magical principle. They guide molar teeth in their eruption patterns and help them assume favorable positions that improve the relationship between the upper and lower jaws.

Still a trickle of interest in this approach is beginning to flow in America. Viken Sassouni, a Lebanese educated in France where he was trained in the use of activators, has been head of the orthodontic department at the University of Pittsburgh since the late 1960's. He has been quietly introducing this suspect European technique into his clinic and, very cautiously, begun to publish his results. He knows that the American orthodontic establishment, when it is not actively hostile to activators, is, at best, indifferent. Therefore, in March, 1972, he wrote prudently that by using functional methods " . . . it is possible to alter the position of the mandible . . . " But as for the crucial question, whether or not, "orthopedic forces" could stimulate extra growth, he hedged. " . . . We must still be reserved," he said.[10] In a course on activators given to practicing orthodontists a year later, he indicated that he would soon be prepared to make more positive claims.[11] European advocates of activator treatment are not so hesitant. Professor Maurice Reboul, head of the orthodontic department at the University of Marseille, who helped Sassouni teach the course, is convinced that activators can cause the deposition of bone, on the head of the condyle, a feat that most American experts are about as ready to accept as the news that someone has learned how to square the circle. Reboul insists that the activator can be an effective addition to an orthodontist's bag of tools, no matter where he practices, but warns that it must be used only in carefully selected cases. Too many French dentists try to use the activator for everything, he told a friend in the spring of 1973. In the hands of such diagnostic dullards, Reboul said dramatically, the activator can often produce real *catastrophes*. After all, he continued, there is a great difference between what activators can do and what fixed appliances can do. Each has its place. Then he said, with the special impish charm that is as native to the sweet soil of southern France as vineyards, "Vive la différence!" Or at least he should have. His friend's recollection is a trifle unclear on that point.[12]

Chapter Fourteen

THE ROLE OF SURGERY IN ORTHODONTICS, PAST, PRESENT, AND FUTURE

> Unfortunately there were occasions when in his anxiety not to drop the ball out of his mouth while flinging off his glove, he would take it too far back between his molars, and find himself unable to extricate it unassisted. It happened infrequently, but always in the same tense situation; with the same disastrous result; an inside-the-mouth grand-slam home run.
>
> Philip Roth, *The Great American Novel.*

The science of oral surgery has made great strides since the World War II days when one-armed Bud Parusha tried to play right field for the old Port Ruppert Mundys of Philip Roth's glorious Patriot League. Still it's unlikely that even the most sophisticated of present day operative techniques could have helped Parusha much in mastering the unique hand-to-mouth style he had of pegging the ball into home plate. Sometimes he failed altogether because of a tragic flaw in his "strong bite." He had worked hard to perfect that bite "over the years by five minutes of chewing on a tennis ball before going to sleep each night." Could a 1973 surgical repair have given his tempero-mandibular joint the extra maneuverability Parusha yearned for? We'll never know.

But there can be no question whatever that oral surgeons who already do much to help improve bites and correct other orthodontic defects will surely do even more in the years ahead. First, of course, their help is needed for extractions. Orthodontists neither fill nor remove teeth: when they announce their specialization they limit their practices to straightening teeth—nothing more. There are two good practical reasons for this act of renunciation. First, the acquisition of true understanding of and competence in the field demands a reasonable amount of concentration. Second, relations with the so-called "referring doctors" would surely deteriorate if orthodontists were thought of as competitors. This means that all orthodontic patients continue to be supervised by their family dentists. Not only will the dentist be on the lookout for cavities or other calamities but he can also cast an appraising eye on the appliances to see that they are not threatening the health of teeth or gums. When extractions are needed the family dentist can do them. Sometimes, however, he may decline the honor either because minor oral surgery is not a field that ordinarily interests him or because the individual case may be too complicated for him to cope with comfortably. Also, the removal of four bicuspid teeth, so frequently required for the smooth unraveling of intertwined incisors, is not something a general dentist is usually equipped to do in a single sitting. And this may be just what an apprehensive patient requires.

So the oral surgeon, another specialist, is called upon. By using general anaesthesia, he can extract four teeth, one from each quadrant of the mouth, in a single visit, instead of easing out two the first week and two the second week, as the family dentist would do. While oral surgeons can thus avoid a duplication or dragging out of what has to be, at least to some extent, an emotionally trying proceeding, a new element of risk is introduced. Why use a potent general anaesthetic when something simpler will do? For although the safety record for general anaesthesia in dental offices is high, it deals with the central nervous system while local anaesthesia, by definition, numbs not the mind but a small and restricted part of the body. But general anaesthesia is convenient. It avoids the "needle" which terrifies many children. And it makes it possible for four bicuspids to be removed at once, something that conventional dental wisdom insists is not possible with a local anaesthetic. In order to do it effectively some oral surgeons are using newer pharmocological methods that put patients into a deep state of relaxation but do not abolish reflexes or induce the kind of muscular loss of control that accompanies traditional general anaesthetics. These modern agents, variously called sedatives or sedanalgesics, can be adroitly combined with locally injected chemicals, like xylocaine, so as to allay fear and apprehension while at the same time lowering risks considerably.

It is even possible, by using a technique that is called, aptly enough, infiltration, to numb both jaws sufficiently with nothing but local anaesthesia for the removal of four teeth at once. Afterwards the mouth is not left so frozen that the patient feels excessively uncomfortable. So here is still one more issue for thoughtful parents to consider. Is it better to have extractions performed all at once while the patient has been carried into a light level of unconsciousness by medication usually injected into the arm or should the operation be done by numbing the jawbones either at one sitting or in two visits? Which technique will cause greater psychological trauma? Though it is certain that local anaesthetics are safer than general agents, is the difference really significant? Would a psychosedative be appropriate? Or some combination approach? The fact is that each child has unique emotional, physical, and dental requirements. There is no reason why the interested parties—patients, parents, and dentists—can't talk it over to see what route best suits each child from every standpoint.

An oral surgeon's services can also be required when teeth fail to erupt properly. Sometimes they are prevented from coming into place by a physical obstruction, like a supernumerary tooth. But sometimes they stray from home base for no apparent reason. If there is little likelihood the tooth will erupt of its own free will, an oral surgeon may be asked to uncover the reluctant tooth or teeth; that is to remove any gingiva and bone that lie between it and the oral cavity. Sometimes this provision of a clear channel will be all that is needed for resumption of an interrupted journey into the dental arch. Other teeth may be so far out of line that the orthodontist will want to hook them into his appliance in order to apply direct pressure to the erring brethren. (In cases like this, the new bonding techniques can be most helpful, especially if the surgeon is only able to uncover a small portion of the unerupted tooth.) There are some instances, happily rare, in which very little can be done to retrieve a strayed tooth. It may be ankylosed, physically joined to the surrounding bone and as unwilling to budge as Martin Luther or it may be in such an inaccessible position that any attempt to recover it would be more trouble than it was worth. Such teeth may be suitable candidates for extraction.

Oral surgeons are also called upon to help out by removing frenii. Despite the classical sound of it, this does not mean they are asked to join Caesar in suppressing some dissident tribe in Northern Gaul. The prosaic fact is that the cutting away of a thick tissue attachment, a frenum, between teeth, usually central incisors, can often facilitate the closing of spaces. Not infrequently the maxillary frenum is too large or too tightly attached and appears to cause or contribute to the maintainance of an unsightly gap between anterior teeth. As Dougherty remarked in a 1971 issue of the Journal of the American Dental Association, "most orthodontists agree that space closure of the diastema should occur first and the surgical removal of the frenum second."[1] By establishing this sequence of events the practitioner can forestall the unwelcome exchange of a troublesome frenum for an even more irksome band of thick scar tissue. On the mandible, a taut lingual frenum can limit maneuverability of the tongue and thus interfere with swallowing or talking. Excessively tense labial frenii may pull gingival tissue away from anterior teeth and threaten, like a wronged woman, to expose all, in this case root surface, not intimate romantic details. Operations for the removal of frenii need to be done carefully, of course, but they are minor and do not usually call for hospitalization.

While these kinds of surgical assistance are important, they remain secondary. But since standard orthodontic treatment is not only occasionally painful but can also be painfully slow, sooner or later somebody had to wonder if things couldn't be speeded up a bit with the swift stroke of a scalpel. As far back as 1849, S. P. Hullihen of Wheeling in what was then still Virginia, performed the first known mandibular resection to correct a prognathism and open bite which had been aggravated by tissue damage suffered in a fire. Angle, who was familiar with Hullihen's work, referring particularly to the splint the Virginian used to hold the separated parts of the jaw together during healing, apparently did not consider that Hullihen had set a precedent. When he wrote about dento-facial orthopedic surgery in his 6th edition of 1900, Angle never mentioned his predecessor's pioneering efforts. He began his account of the revolutionary jaw operation with these words:

> While all tooth movement is essentially surgical that by the use of appliances may be properly called Conservative Surgery. To distinguish the more bold or aggressive operations involving the use of cutting instruments we will designate them as Operative Surgery. While such operations should probably be employed only as auxiliary to the conservative method, they are doubtless destined to play a more important part in the practice of the future . . .

Angle's prophecy has been borne out strikingly in recent years. This is how he described his original work at the time: "Several years ago the author became convinced that no operation depending upon tooth movement alone could establish the facial lines in certain cases of pronounced overdevelopment of the mandible. It seemed to him," Angle continued, delicately referring to himself in the third person, "that such cases might be successfully treated by the removal of a section of bone" from each side of the jaw. "The author's proposition," he went on, "was discussed with surgeons and dentists. A few of the former believed it to be practicable: the latter almost invariably predicted certain failure. Since first proposed the operation has been performed twice—once successfully . . . in St. Louis . . . and once in New Orleans, when it nearly cost the patient his life, with the total loss of the mandible through necrosis." [2] It would seem that the pessimistic dentists and the optimistic surgeons were each half right. Since those bold pioneering days, the odds on a successful outcome for a mandibular resection, as the operation is called, have improved considerably. It isn't even necessary to journey to St. Louis to have the job done properly. But surgical reduction of a large jaw is still reserved for extreme cases where simple orthodontic means have already failed or are deemed to be inadequate. (See figure 13.)

What should be done when a young child shows an anterior cross bite that might be either a modest malalignment of teeth, which would respond well to standard orthodontic treatment, or could be just the beginning of a severe jaw problem that would defy even the most astute appliance manipulation? For the first category braces are just what the doctor ordered. For the second, they are really a waste of time; in the long run only surgery can help. But even so, it's generally best to try the "conservative" treatment first because there is no reliable way of predict-

The Role of Surgery in Orthodontics

ing which anterior cross bites will involve misplaced teeth alone and which will go on growing into true mandibular prognathism. In that 1971 issue of the Journal of the American Dental Association devoted to surgical orthodontics, Donald Poulton wrote that, "Some patients who have mild class III problems at the age of 12 years get no worse, others who start with a Class II relationship develop severe Class III problems." Still others, he pointed out, whose skeletal dimensions appeared to be within normal limits at age 12 will begin to have "distinctly Class III facial appearance . . . by age 14 . . . Three years later the anterior teeth may be in cross bite relationship . . . In spite of any orthodontic efforts." [3]

The parent whose child has endured substantial orthodontic attention but whose remorseless mandibular growth has propelled him by the close of puberty directly into the hands of an oral surgeon may ask, Poulton says, "whether the orthodontic treatment accomplished any useful purpose." Poulton doesn't dare speculate what the patient himself may think of all this but goes directly on to answer his hypothetical question. "It is probable," he says, "that . . . the treatment lessened the severity of the problem." [4] Well, maybe. But such "lessened severity" neither simplifies the eventual operation nor improves its outcome. In any case, it is an idle argument. Parents and orthodontists have no choice. They really have to seize the main chance and select early orthodontic treatment. Most of the time it will work. And no one can tell in advance which times it won't. "This world is not one in which certainty is possible," Bertrand Russell said. We must, he advised, "Act [on the basis of] probabilities . . . with vigor . . ." [5]

The principle that ought to be followed here greatly resembles the law of parsimony which governs the formulation of scientific theories: accept for a working hypothesis the simplest explanation that fits the known facts. Don't look for the most exciting, the most exotic, or even the one that appears to be the most promising. Just work with the most parsimonious theory until new data comes along that dictates a revision.

In attempting to account for its evident stability the ancient Hindus embraced the view that the world rested on a giant elephant. Incorrect, perhaps, but admirable in its parsimony. Unfortunately, the Hindus were not content with this spare contention. They embellished it. The elephant, they said, was standing on an enormous tortoise. If, according to Russell's account of the matter, they were asked, "How about the tortoise?" they replied, "suppose we change the subject." This is the kind of trap that awaits the careless investigator who abandons the law of parsimony.

A prudent receiver of health services ought to reason in the same way: accept the simplest, least dangerous treatment that will do the job. If teeth can be straightened with braces, that should be the method of choice, not a dramatic operation, which may be quicker, but as Angle discovered, can have its complications. Of course, the progress of traditional orthodontic care can also be mined with hazards as will be seen in the next chapter. But actually, an *either or* decision between orthodontics and surgery rarely comes up. One American surgeon put it this way, "Surgery is not a substitute for good orthodontic practice but a supplement and alternative when conservative possibilities for correction are limited." [6] Generally speaking, orthodontic forces can reposition only teeth and the bone immediately surrounding them, the alveolar bone, except when clever treatment timing joins with growth to bring about an improvement in the relationship between the mandible and the maxilla. If major movement of bones is required, surgical methods, or possibly dento-facial orthopedics, must be enlisted.

Similar considerations of parsimony might persuade a couple to control family size by using mechanical devices instead of pills that could interfere with the body's hormonal balance or even lead to unpleasant side effects. And when it comes to tooth extractions, why take the slight risk of general anaesthesia when local anaesthesia is even less threatening? This kind of parsimony, although it is occasionally expensive in dollars, should have a strong appeal to people everywhere.[7]

Of course, surgical safety standards are much higher now than they were in Angle's day. And there are some attractive arguments for adopting a surgical approach for the correction of a facial deformity instead of submitting to long term orthodontic care: not only is an operation swifter, it can also do things that could never be achieved even with the most ingenious array of wires and hooks. An open bite that might never respond to orthodontic force can be closed right up surgically just as closed bites can be immediately unlocked. Enormous bony protrusions, of either jaw, can be eliminated in hours, not years, with knife and suture. In other words, while orthodontists can now proudly assert that they have the capability of moving any tooth in any direction, or plane of space, as they like to put it, oral surgeons can almost literally do the same thing with the jaw bones themselves. This is exactly what the adherents of heavy orthopedic force are attempting to do. So far it is not clear whether or not they will have the same degree of success that the surgeons seem to be gaining.

Although the surgical correction of mandibular prognathisms began, as we saw, with Hullihen more than 120 years ago, other malocclusions resisted the surgeon's scalpel until Cohn-Stock, in Europe, in 1921, attempted to reduce a severe maxillary protrusion in the operating room. The condition regressed within six months. But by the early 1960's the technique had improved so dramatically that patients were hurrying from all over the world to Zurich, Switzerland, where Professor Hugo Obwegeser, Chief of the Dental Institute of the University of Zurich was skillfully executing almost every conceivable variety of maxillo-facial operation. American surgeons have also been making pilgrimages to Zurich to learn from Obwegeser much as psychiatrists flocked to Vienna fifty years ago to study with Freud. MacIntosh, an American advocate of Obwegeser's techniques, writes that "possibilities in alveolar arch surgery are nearly limitless." [8]

Cy Amato, one of the American surgeons who has made the trip to Zurich, puts it this way, "The advent of newer drugs, instruments and materials has made it possible to apply standard surgical principles to the correction of cranio-facial deformities. The essence of maxillo-facial or orthodontic surgery is to identify the deformity using cephalometric methods, section the malpositioned bone or bones, place them in correct position, and secure the fragments for six to eight weeks to allow healing in this new position." [9]

This approach to facial deformities is not designed to move individual teeth but to restore harmony to the function and appearance of the bones of the face by moving segments of bone which may contain three to six teeth or the whole jaw, upper or lower, containing all of the teeth. In rare instances the complete face from below the eyes to and including the upper jaw may be moved.

The possible variations are many and require an active imagination on the part of the surgeon. Most conditions can be treated by surgery performed from within the mouth eliminating the possibility of unsightly scars. The postoperative discomfort is minimal, many times relieved by aspirin.

This is a new and exciting area of dentistry and surgery that will find an important place in the treatment of facial deformities. Often these dramatic improvements must be preceded not only by orthodontic planning but also by some preliminary treatment. In some cases, additional orthodontic care is required to tuck all the loose ends into place.

As orthodontics moves along into the 1970's, there can be little doubt that the surgical contribution to the resolution of facial deformities will increase. At the same time stronger and less conspicuous attachments will surely make orthodontic treatment more palatable than it now is to reluctant adolescents. Whether or not the still sputtering trend toward dento-facial orthopedics will achieve the same accelerating pace is a matter open to considerable question. There are other unanswered questions that impede the steady forward stride of orthodontics. We'll examine them more closely in the next chapter and then try to lighten the blow with a heady look at some even wilder possibilities whose implications are just beginning to be examined.

Chapter Fifteen

CALCULATED RISKS AND RISKY CALCULATIONS

> Mentir comme un arracheur de dents.
>
> (To lie like a puller of teeth)
> French idiomatic expression

"Belle continuously probed and picked at her lower left premolars for almost 30 minutes." Quite an extended period to devote to care of the teeth. And unusual, extremely unusual. For, at eight, Belle is considerably younger than the average orthodontic patient who, unlike Belle, is continually bombarded with exhortations to keep his mouth spotless and rarely does. But Belle is not an orthodontic patient at all. She is a chimpanzee, observed, never exhorted, at the Delta Regional Primate Research Center of Tulane University. Belle and her buddies, McGrew and Tutin reported in the *Journal of the American Dental Association,* "inspect, clean, and extract their own and each other's teeth."[1] Many human patients seem much less devoted to the principles of sound oral hygiene than their simian cousins, exhibiting a dental version of "la belle indifférence" which gravely threatens the smooth course of orthodontic progress. If food particles are allowed to accumulate around the edges of orthodontic bands the eventual result will be decalcification of the enamel. This means that ugly white marks can be left on teeth no matter how well appliances are made. And, worse still, if bands cease to fit properly, if some obscure edge loses its tight contact with the tooth it covers, food can wedge in between metal and tooth and create even deeper lesions. That's why orthodontist, family dentist, and patient should work together to make sure bands continue to fit tightly and are kept reasonably clean. When direct bonding of attachments to tooth surfaces becomes commonplace these pesky foods traps will disappear along with the metallic glint of a full set of bands. So revised cementation techniques will be one method for reducing the risks that accompany sloppy oral hygiene. Improved motivational programs stressing, perhaps, appropriate rewards, may be another. One puckish observer (well, me, actually) has suggested that a good way to encourage young people to keep their teeth clean would be to make toothbrushing illegal.

In addition to the harm that may befall the hard parts of the dental crown, the surrounding soft tissues of the mouth can also be insulted by orthodontic efforts, particularly in a chronically dirty mouth. Inflamed gums all too often tag along after the installation of a new set of braces as closely as the little lamb followed Mary. Sometimes gums become so sore and puffy that orthodontic treatment must stop until order is restored to the mutinous tissues. This may call for only a little simple treatment but the situation could become serious enough to require removal of appliances until health returns to the area.

Other things can also go wrong during orthodontic treatment. Even the fundamental principle upon which tooth movement depends may suddenly and inexplicably suspend itself. When force is applied to a tooth the usual and expected response is for the adjacent bone politely to accede to pressure, melt, thaw, and resolve itself into a dew, thereby allowing the tooth to move into the vacuum which, it is well known, Nature abhors. But on some occasions the root surface is absorbed, too. The orthodontist who all along had been expecting from this outer root covering the steadfast behavior of Benedict Arnold on the Plains of Abraham, finds instead he has to deal with the traitor of West Point. The treacherous roots of the teeth of some patients occasionally fail to demonstrate grace under orthodontic pressure and shrink, literally as well as figuratively. Most of the time the physical loss is minimal and of little importance. But it can be severe. When he recognizes the presence of root resorption, or shortening, an orthodontist may decide the time has come to leave well enough alone and call a halt to the proceedings. How can he tell whether the pressures his appliances exert are producing smooth and steady results unmarred by unwelcome side effects or, instead, are causing trouble? Easy. He takes checkup X-rays. He knows what the teeth looked like to start with because he took diagnostic films and can make the needed comparison. All very good. All very prudent, professional, and beneficial. Well, not entirely.

Man has always lived under a faint, imperceptible drizzle of atomic radiation which pours down steadily from the cosmos. Only within the last 80 years has he learned to add his own contribution to this shower, thus unlocking the mysteries of the human skeleton, including its jawbones and teeth, and leveling Nagasaki in the process . Until recently he has been reluctant to admit to himself that the results of this ceaseless downpour are cumulative—they do not fade away in time—and that even the peacetime bombardment is harmful. Whenever a government agency releases a report on the effects of ionizing radiation it lowers its suggested "maximum permissible dose" downward. There are two types of dangers posed by all atomic radiation: one is to the exposed individual who runs increased risks of contracting certain diseases and the other is the possible creation of harmful traits that will be passed on to future generations. Young patients are especially vulnerable on both counts. Their tissues are particularly susceptible to radiation effects and, of course, their breeding years all lie ahead. The 469 page document released in November, 1972, by a special committee of the National

Academy of Sciences-National Research Council was no exception to the rule that things looked grimmer when they were more closely examined. The report warned, according to the *New York Times*, that "excess deaths and illnesses accompanied increases in the national level of radiation exposure." [2] Apart from natural background radiation upon which not even an act of Congress can have the slightest effect, medical and dental X-rays now account for the largest part of this exposure.

The committee discreetly commented, again as reported by the *Times*, that in the area of "diagnostic radiation . . . there is room for improvement." [3] Conscientious practitioners who are well aware of the need for self regulation in radiography already take every known precaution. They reduce radiation by special techniques that include the use of filters, screening devices, and protective lead aprons and limit their picture taking to instances of clear need. There is, of course, a risk of erring too far in the direction of caution. By omitting a potentially informative film because he is concerned about the dangers of radiation an orthodontist can miss signs of decay or other dental disease, plan his treatment along erroneous lines, or, if he has started out correctly, be led astray into some damaging detour. X-rays have a respected and useful role to play in orthodontics, as they do in many branches of medicine but a prudent parent will not be stepping out of line if he tells his orthodontist that while he appreciates the need for diagnostic films he hopes they are being taken with the utmost regard for safety standards. The marvelous tool of X-rays must be used with infinite respect and care. Here, yet again the orthodontist has to steer a painstaking course between the Scylla of too much of one thing and the Charybydis of too little of the other. He seems, in fact, so incessantly to be required to maneuver delicately between reef and sandbar that he might be well advised to spend his spare time taking a course, not in the latest technique for bending wires, but in yachting.

Occasionally during treatment some patients, usually females, develop clicking sounds when they close their jaws. The noises, sometimes as loud as a muffled rifle shot, come from the place where the mandible meets the skull, the temporomandibular joint (TMJ). Not only can this joint become rowdy, it can also become painful. Similar symptoms can also arise, of course, elsewhere in the body but presumably under different circumstances. There is a possibility that orthodontic treatment itself, especially the use of elastics hooked from one jaw to another, may contribute to this disorder but only in the TMJ, not in the hip. No one is really quite sure, however. In fact, of all the disputes that swirl about dental issues the one focussed on trouble in the temporomandibular joint may well be the most confusing. To illustrate the tangled nature of the controversy, which is not without its comic aspects, the following authoritative explanations of TMJ disease have been paraphrased as concisely and as fairly as possible. They all appeared in the July, 1969 issue of the *Journal of the American Dental Association* which was devoted to "Derangements of the Temporomandibular Joint":

- Psychological factors are the chief cause of TMJ disturbances.[4]

- The percentage of adults suffering from TMJ problems who have crooked teeth proves that malocclusion is the chief cause of TMJ disturbances.[5]

- Despite the emphasis previously placed on crooked teeth as the cause of TMJ disturbances, many patients with malocclusion do *not* develop these problems.[6]

- The inadequate explanation provided by the "tooth theories" ultimately led to "tooth muscle" theories which were better but failed to answer other criticisms. It is our belief that muscle spasm is the primary factor responsible for TMJ disturbances.[7]

- Crooked teeth should be classified as a predisposing cause of TMJ disturbances: teeth clenching, bruxism, or other occlusal use and abuse would be the activating cause.[8]

- Poor function of the masticatory and cervical muscles causes TMJ disturbances. Symptoms and pain can be controlled by careful grinding of teeth to improve the bite.[9]

- (And from the *American Journal of Orthodontics*, December, 1972.) Informed orthodontists will avoid traditional but irrational methods for the relief of symptoms and the control of pain in TMJ disturbances, such as the grinding of teeth to improve the bite.[10]

All of which *does* seem to prove that no one yet knows *what* causes disturbances of the temporomandibular joint nor what to do about them. (Of course, the possibility that arthritic changes or even a tumor are present must be considered and ruled out before any purely dental treatment is begun.) The fact is that each of the differing, and sometimes directly contradictory, methods of management seem to achieve some "cures." This may confirm the suspicion of one group of investigators that psychological factors do, indeed, underlie most of the painful symptoms which, consequently, respond favorably to any supportive, placebo-type of ministrations. It also seems clear that there is some connection between orthodontic treatment, particularly with inter-maxillary rubber bands, and joint *sounds* if not joint *pains*. (Many people have noisy joints but aren't troubled by them.) Just what the connection is or how frequently it is likely to come up remain mysteries.

Perhaps the most persistent and distressing of the traps that lurk in the path of the orthodontic voyager are the twin calamities of choice of the wrong plan before treatment begins and relapse after it is completed. The traveler may begin his journey toward the distant goal of straight and shining teeth and never reach it because he was headed in the wrong direction. (Teeth, for example, may have been extracted when they shouldn't have been or vice versa.) Or he may finally grasp the prized objective only to watch it slip slowly away. These disasters can be caused by failure to discern the real nature of the problem, they may come about because the patient-doctor team didn't act out an essentially satisfactory scenario with sufficient skill and zeal, or they may result from the fact that the original problem was too severe to be correctable by ordinary orthodontic means. This last category could be a type of mis-diagnosis or it could stem from a vagary in growth that was simply unpredictable.

If only, many an orthodontist has speculated, it *were* possible to know in advance how each patient would grow, respond to treatment or resist it, and to what extent he would cooperate, it might be possible to select a reasonable and appropriate treatment plan for each case. By using a 20th century crystal ball a wary orthodontist might be able to sidestep the snares of root resorption, decalcification, and gingival irritation that are poised to ambush him. If that elusive crystal ball is not yet available in the nation's supply houses, the same electronic marvels that put a man on the moon *are* ready to supply similar services. Computers programmed with suitable orthodontic data, we are told, are capable of unravelling the puzzling dilemmas of malocclusion. In 1969 the first diagnostic cephalometric system was offered to a doubting dental public by the Rocky

Mountain Company, a pioneer orthodontic supply house. "We can say," claimed Robert Ricketts, one of the chief advocates of the program, "with reasonable assurance that the forecasting of growth and behavior is possible both in the short and the long range . . . Cephalometrics, when computerized, becomes the most powerful tool of information yet devised for the practicing orthdontist." [11] How is this scientific triumph going to be perfected? Viken Sassouni, Professor of Orthodontics at the University of Pittsburgh, envisions it this way, "It is possible to install a computer terminal in every dental office. The practitioner would consult the central computer bank and would decide if his plan and that of the main office coincide." Already the diagnostic service established by Sassouni includes 2000 cases and has 720 treatment plans to choose from.[12] Without giving exact figures for his system Ricketts asserts that "storage of data made possible by computerization . . . offers the orthodontist an opportunity to compare his case or group of cases to an atlas of normal growth." [13]

This type of thinking has been attacked by less clinically oriented scientists, like the anatomist Melvin Moss[14] who criticizes orthodontists for their estrangement from the mainstream of anatomical and anthropological research. Orthodontic formulas for evaluating skull shape and size are based on arbitrary landmarks, they say, that have little, if any, relationship to the actual processes of human growth. According to one European scientist, "So far as parts of the head have been studied, it can be concluded that a general direction or rate of growth does not exist."[14a]

Ernie Hixon's disdain for efforts to predict individual development was even sharper: " . . . biologic principles which govern growth of the dentition" he said "are not and cannot be well described by a cephalometric analysis with any better accuracy than archangels describe the paths of the planets." [15] Alton Moore, Professor of Orthodontics at the University of Washington, commented soberly, "Desirable as prediction is from the standpoint of the clinician, no method has as yet been devised to make accurate prediction of future growth a reality. It is true that faces tend to have an individual growth direction and that this direction is relatively constant throughout the growth period. But if this is true, why the need for a systematic analysis to tell us so? The clinician's problems are those persons whose facial growth patterns vary from the usual and whose faces grow in an unfavorable way, varying from the norm, and thus are not predictable, at least not as yet. I sincerely hope that some day I will have to eat these words, but I cannot be optimistic about computerizing biology." [16]

Whether the noble effort to reduce the agonies of diagnostic decisions to a computer's printout is doomed to remain pure balderdash as Hixon thought or is already virtually at hand as Ricketts insists, keeping the ketchup handy for Dr. Moore, we cannot say. The future no doubt holds the answer. That prediction, at least, is a safe one.

Yet another intriguing possibility may or may not lie ahead. Like computerized prediction, its various merits and perils have already begun to stir acrimonious debate in the pages of the orthodontic journals. In May, 1972, J. A. Salzmann, a former president of the American Association of Orthodontists and a prolific writer, broached for the first time the prospect of a technological advance that could deal with malocclusion not by surgery for the late adolescent or adult, not by standard care of twelve year olds, not even by so-called early treatment of eight year olds, but by eliminating the defect with *really* early treatment, before birth.[17]

The breathtaking horizons hinted at by Salzmann lead us to a consideration of the genetic pool, that priceless sea in which are stored up all the myriad traits, characteristics, and even hopes of mankind. Each of us carries in every cell of his body a detailed blueprint for the whole individual. Each trait, for eye color, for jaw size, for tooth position, for all of what we are, is encoded in a gene. The genes, of which there are many thousands, are contained in the chromosomes. For humans the number of chromosomes (the diploid number) carried in the central part—the nucleus—of every body cell is 46. The sex cells, eggs in females and spermatozoa in males, possess just half, 23, the haploid figure. So, when an egg is fertilized and the diploid number restored, each parent contributes half of the total number of chromosomes and thus shares equally in providing the heritage of the offspring. All of the genes of a population together make up its genetic pool, its potential for the future. Genes can be changed by radiation, among other things. These alterations, or mutations, by means of which evolution has thus far progressed, are usually harmful. That is the risk posed to posterity by excessive radiation: it can cause mutations and thereby degrade the genetic pool.

Molecular biologists are slowly unraveling the mysteries of the cell nucleus with its gene-bearing chromosomes which are made up, they have discovered, of nucleic acid, in the form of either ribonucleic acid (RNA) or deoxynucleic acid (DNA). They are even learning how to manipulate these compounds, a capability that has striking implications. Mankind is on the threshold of being able to mastermind its own evolution.[18]

H. J. Muller, an American winner, of the Nobel prize for medicine, in 1946, made the first proposal for direct control of human evolution, which had heretofore depended entirely on capricious and generally deleterious chance mutations. To an assemblage of human geneticists convened in Chicago in September, 1966, Muller suggested that outstanding males, chosen for their moral, physical, and

Calculated Risks and Risky Calculations 131

emotional excellence, should make deposits in the sperm bank. Later, volunteer mothers could select their stand-in mates from a catalogue enumerating the qualifications and specifications of the assorted donors who would remain anonymous and, in all likelihood, have been dead for at least twenty years.[19] Their sperm, of course, would have remained very much alive, frozen like Keats' Grecian lovers of whom he said, "She cannot fade, though thou hast not thy bliss/ For ever wilt thou love, and she be fair." Thanks to this technique, average parents, like you and me, could enrich their own lacklustre genetic qualities with an infusion drawn from the most splendid specimens mankind has produced, taking care, of course, to rule out any Shakespeares or Newtons or Freuds with crooked teeth. Despite the technical feasibility of this scheme, there has been no headlong rush to implement it, for several good reasons. For one thing, we have as yet only the dimmest inkling of how many genes there are, what signals turn them on or off, and the action of all but a small number of them. So an estimate of the true breeding value of any man, even an Einstein, would be mere guesswork. And even if the plan did produce superior infants as it surely would most of the time, its radical and bizarre connotations might be the final blow in the destruction of the family.

Another startling suggestion was made by F.H.C. Crick who, with J.D. Watson, won the Nobel prize for partially breaking the genetic code with the discovery of the double helix formula for DNA. Crick speculated, in 1962, that it would soon be possible, using methods already known, to supply an oral contraceptive to entire populations by adding an inhibiting substance to foods or liquids. Then only those prospective parents deemed to be eugenically fit would be issued the antidote that would permit conception.[20] This scheme might speedily weed out substandard genes but its anti-democratic features are so blatant that they scarcely require comment. Luckily, Crick's curious proposal has been steadfastly ignored.

Some possibilities, on the other hand, are beginning to attract lavish attention. They are so wild that even Buck Rogers, the comic strip hero from the 25th century, would scorn them on the ground they were too fantastic. But cloning, the exact duplication of one individual after another after another—as though they were turned out by a printing press—is already feasible with animals as high on the evolutionary scale as frogs. How is this done? Simple. One merely removes the nucleus of a fertilized egg with a micro-pipette or inactivates it with ultra-violet rays, and substitutes the nucleus of a cell plucked from the individual one wishes to Xerox. Thus, the chromosomes and their genes provided by the true parents are replaced with a set donated by the false parent. (Nucleii from cells lining the intestine are especially good for this purpose, if you were wondering where to look.) The creature or creatures who will then develop from the altered egg or eggs will mimic in every conceivable way, trait for trait, gene for gene, the "parent" from whose stomach the nucleus was removed. (Whatever aspects of personality, physique, intelligence, and behavior that are controlled by environment will, of course, differ from individual to individual. The general lines of physical appearance and basic capacity will not.) Scientists have little doubt that they will soon be able to "clone" cattle. Somewhere between the years 2020 and 2030 it will probably be possible to construct exact replicas of human beings. This may be the answer to the great people crisis that began with Adam and Eve or it might just be the start of more trouble.

What has all this got to do with orthodontics? The answer to that question is simple, too. The possibility of cranking out a precise copy of a Mozart or an Elvis Presley as easily as Ellsberg Xeroxed the Pentagon Papers is real, not a hallucination. It lies scarcely 50 years in the future. The day when less spectacular tinkering with genetic programming becomes practical may be closer. Marshall Nirenberg, a leading biochemical geneticist, has said that, "Genetic surgery, applied to micro-organisms, is a reality. I have little doubt that the obstacles will eventually be overcome. The only question is when. My guess is that cells will be programmed with synthesized messages within 25 years. If efforts along these lines were intensified, bacteria might be programmed within five years."

"The point which deserves special emphasis," Nirenberg added, according to Gordon Taylor writing in *The Biological Time Bomb,* "is that man may be able to program his own cells with synthesized information long before he will be able to assess adequately the long-term consequences of such alterations, long before he will be able to formulate goals, and long before he can resolve the ethical and moral problems which will be raised." Edward Tatum optimistically predicted, according to Taylor, that the day would come when new genes or gene products could be slipped into the cells of defective organs.[21] If Mommy and Daddy were careless enough to handicap you with an enormous lower jaw or buck teeth, some friendly scientist could remedy the error by changing genes while you were in the womb. Inept fathers who can't even change *diapers* ought to be suitably impressed. Dr. Salzmann, however, is evidently not overawed by the technical virtuosity that the feat will require nor is he intimidated by doubts about its social value.[22]

Other geneticists, like Professor D. Klein, of the University of Geneva, aren't worried about the moral implications of "genetic engineering" either, but for a different reason. They just don't think it can really be done. "We possess," Klein says, "neither the knowledge nor the wisdom necessary for the establishment of the kind of program of 'genetic engineering' certain biologists [and orthodontists] are predicting." [23]

This cautious view is shared by Samuel Pruzansky, director of the Center for Craniofacial Anomalies at the University of Illinois. He caustically condemned the type of "exuberant, Promethean predictions of unlimited control" that led Salzmann to refer to the ". . . aborting of harmful genes, and the introduction of desirable genes into the early forming embryos. These techniques eventually will make possible the prevention of many antenatal, congenital, and postnatal genetically induced dentofacial anomalies, including dental malocclusion." Pruzansky's letter attacking Salzmann's exalted vision of the future cited the opposition of Friedmann and Roblin, of the Salk Institute for Biological Studies, to "further attempts at gene therapy in human patients for the foreseeable future." Efforts to replace "defective" DNA with "good" DNA should be postponed, if not abandoned entirely, because our understanding of genetic disease remains "rudimentary" and "we have no information on the short-range and long-term side effects of gene therapy," Pruzansky said, summing up the Friedmann-Roblin position.[24] Anyhow, if this kind of truly early treatment ever does get started it will be directed initially against the relatively few disorders that can be traced to a single gene. The shape, size, and growth patterns of facial structures are considered to be under the control of many genes. Despite the tricky things that are being done to frogs in laboratories nowadays, human beings, it seems, are likely to require the services of orthodontists, working postnatally, for a very long time to come.

If this is so, an informed public will still have to interest itself in the humdrum details of how and why errant teeth are moved from one place to another. Why? Thomas Szasz, the iconoclastic psychiatrist who considers mental illness to be a myth, addressed himself to this question in a recent interview with Paul Kurtz in the *Humanist* magazine. Doesn't the public, Kurtz asked, need to be protected from "incompetent . . . practitioners?"

"Oh, I agree that people *need* protection," Szasz answered. But, he added, ". . . This is a vastly complicated problem for which there are no simple solutions. The first line of protection for the public lies, I would say, in self protection. People must learn to grow up and learn to protect themselves—or suffer the consequences."

How are they to do this? Through education. "Why do you think that people don't know more about medicine?" Kurtz asked.

"There are many reasons for that. One is because they aren't taught anything about it . . . most professions thrive on mystification; on keeping the public in the dark—despite all the protestations about popularizing medical knowledge. I have always thought that 12- and 13-year-olds could be taught a great deal about how the body works—really works; it's no more difficult either to teach or learn that than is algebra or French grammar." [25]

This is really the crucial point. There are no simple answers: none for the practitioner striving to select the most suitable course of action from a bewildering array of alternatives, none for the parent and patient trying to make their way through unfamiliar territory. And since there is absolutely no algebra in this book and only a soupçon of French grammar, it may provide a useful map for a confused traveler.[26]

GLOSSARY

ACTIVATOR—A large, removable device into which the lower teeth can bite in only one, predetermined position. It is supposed to retrain reflex jaw muscle patterns so that the "bite" will be improved.

ANCHORAGE—The relatively stable supporting area from which force is applied to move designated teeth. Anchorage can consist of some teeth, all the teeth in a jaw, or the back of the neck or the top of the head. It incorporates the orthodontic version of the lever principle.

ANGLE CLASSIFICATION—E. H. Angle, pioneer American orthodontist (1855-1931), separated dental irregularities into three categories: Class I—the two jaws meet properly but teeth are crowded or spaced. Class II—The upper protrude with respect to the lower teeth. Division I, the upper anterior teeth are inclined forward; Division 2, the upper anterior teeth tend to be leaning backwards. Class III—The teeth of the lower jaw are too far forward with respect to the upper teeth.

APPLIANCE—Any of the devices designed to move or guide teeth or jaws. They may be (a) fixed—cemented in place, —or, (b) removable and thus worn at the pleasure of the patient.

ARCH—The approximately half moon shape assumed by teeth on the jaw bones. The main regulating wire used in fixed appliances conforms to this pattern and so it is known as an arch wire. It may lie on the tongue side of teeth and be called a lingual arch or be placed on the lip side where it is referred to as a labial arch.

ARTICULATION—A joint, a meeting of two bones. In dentistry, the positioning of teeth and the way teeth of one jaw meet those of the other.

BAND—The collar of thin metal which carries one or more attachments into which an arch wire can be secured. It is fitted carefully and then cemented to a tooth.

BEGG TECHNIQUE—A fixed appliance method introduced by Angle's student, Raymond Begg. Using one of Angle's earlier appiances in a modified form, Begg tips the teeth rapidly toward improved postures and uprights them later.

BEHAVIORISM—The psychological school that considers observable and measurable performance the only valid subject for investigation. Behaviorists either doubt the existance of or are uninterested in unconscious mental processes.

BEHAVIOR MODIFICATION—A psychotherapy based on principles of behaviorism.

BODY IMAGE—A psychoanalytic term meaning simply the picture of our own body which we form in our own mind. Real or imagined defects can have an impact on self esteem far greater than would seem to be warranted by objective standards.

BRACKET—One of the attachments formerly soldered but now ususally welded to the front surface of a band. The arch wire is secured to it in order to transmit the appropriate quantity of force.

BRIDGE—A replacement for a missing tooth. It can be fixed or removable. Fixed bridges, which are thought to be more satisfactory in terms of dental health, require the cutting down of adjacent teeth on at least one but usually both sides of the missing member. The bridge will consist of the false tooth (dummy or pontic), soldered to the crowns which are cemented on the prepared neighboring teeth, the abutments.

Glossary 139

BRUXISM—The habitual grinding or clenching of teeth. This possibly damaging dental behavior often occurs, like snoring, at night, without the patient's knowledge.

BUCCAL—In the direction of the cheeks.

BUTTON—One of the do-hickeys welded onto bands. Buttons are usually placed on the tongue side to serve as fasteners for elastic bands or as a means of tying together recently moved teeth in order to stabilize them.

CANINE—The third tooth from the midline. Strong and sturdy, it can serve as a useful weapon for belligerently inclined animals.

CAP—A disfigured or poorly formed anterior tooth may be appropriately prepared and then covered with a cap or jacket crown, usually made of porcelain, sometimes backed with reinforcing gold.

CARIES—Tooth decay.

CEMENTUM—The calcified tissue, closely resembling bone, that lines the root surfaces of teeth.

CEPHALOMETRICS—The X-Ray system used to study facial skeletons including the teeth and their relationship to jawbones and other surrounding structures. Each film is taken with both source of radiation and patient immobilized in a standardized position. Any variations in succeeding films must, therefore, be due to growth or orthodontic treatment, not changes in placement of patient or X-Ray machine.

CHROMOSOME—The threadlike bodies found in the nucleii of cells. They carry genes.

CLEAT—Like the button, a device for hooking elastics or tying teeth together.

CLEFT PALATE—When the two parts of the maxilla fail to unite an opening or fissure remains in the roof of the mouth.

CLONING—The artificial reproduction of another, identical organism made by nurturing a single cell from the "parent" in an articial non-sexual way.

CONDYLE—The rounded protuberance on a bone. In dentistry, it is the knob atop the ramus of lower jaw. The mandibular condyle articulates with the skull.

CONNECTIVE TISSUE—Like the other major tissue systems of the body, connective tissue is an aggregate of similar cells and cell products forming a distinctive structure. The function of connective tissue is to join together, support, or surround other tissues.

CROWN—Each tooth has a crown. It is the part that appears in the mouth above the gum. When it is defective it can be restored with a gold or synthetic crown.

CUSPID—Another name for canine tooth.

DECALCIFICATION—Loss of any part of the hard surface of a tooth through prolonged contact with food debris and the resultant production of acid.

DECIDUOUS TEETH—The 20 primary teeth, 10 in each jaw, that are replaced by permanent successors.

DEGLUTITION—The act of swallowing sometimes accompanied by exuberant tongue activity that can displace teeth.

DENTIN—The calcified part of the crown of the tooth that lies immediately under the outer covering of enamel.

DENTITION—All of the teeth of an animal, including the human animal, taken together.

Glossary

DESENSITISATION—Sometimes an exposed root surface can become sensitive—to changes in temperature. Application of various ointments may relieve the tenderness. Also, a type of behavior modification designed progressively to reduce phobias or other fears.

DIAGNOSIS—The art or act of recognizing a disease or disorder from its appearance or its symptoms. Also the decision reached in this act.

DIASTEMA—A space between teeth especially between the upper central incisors.

DISHED IN—The unattractive, caved-in look imparted to a face when upper anterior teeth are pushed or tipped too sharply toward the tongue.

DISTAL—The side or position furthest from the center.

EDGEWISE TECHNIQUE—An orthodontic method devised by Angle which requires the banding of many teeth. Precision movements are obtained by the engagement of an edgewise or rectangular wire into tight fitting receptacles (brackets) attached to teeth.

ELASTICS—Small elastic ringlets are attached by patients to hooks, usually one in each jaw, so as to apply force to teeth and thus to move them.

EMBOUCHURE—The way a musical instrument is placed in the mouth (*bouche* in French). Faulty embouchure was once thought to have a harmful effect on tooth position but this is now held to be unlikely.

EPIDEMIOLOGY—The study of widespread diseases or disorders.

EROGENOUS—Sexually gratifying or satisfying. Any area of the body can be an erogenous zone but some more so than others. Even the body itself, taken as a whole, can qualify.

ETCHING—The weakening of the hard surface of a tooth from the long term action of acid developed in areas where food debris piles up because of inadequate tooth brushing. Roughly equivalent to decalcification.

ETIOLOGY—The cause of a disease or disturbance.

EXPANSION—Widening of the dental arches to provide additional space for crooked or protruding teeth.

FIXED APPLIANCE—An orthodontic device that is cemented to teeth.

FRENUM—A fold or membrane that limits the motion of a part. If the maxillary frenum which is attached to the lip comes down too far it can interfere with correct positioning of incisor teeth or contribute to the maintenance of a diastema. A lingual frenum if too tightly attached can interfere with movements of the tongue and indirectly affect tooth alignment.

GENE—The agent for the transmission of inherited characteristics, found on chromosomes.

GENETICS—The science of heredity.

GINGIVA—The gums.

HEAD GEAR—A means of applying force to teeth through elastic straps or rings or springs from an achorage source at the back of the neck or the top of the head. Usually worn at home but sometimes designed for 24 hour a day use.

IMPACTION—A tooth that is tightly wedged by one or more neighbors or whose path of entry into the dental arch it blocked is said to be impacted.

Glossary

INCISAL—In the direction of the biting or cutting edge of an anterior tooth.

INCISOR—An anterior tooth. There are four in each jaw.

JACKET—A cap.

LABIAL—In the direction of the lips.

LATENCY PERIOD—In psychoanalysis, a period in middle childhood from perhaps, five to twelve years, when both sexual and aggressive impulses are thought to be reduced in intensity allowing the child's attention to be directed outward. Educators think latency period children are anxious to learn. They may also be excellent candidates for orthodontic treatment from a psychological point of view.

LEVELING—The bringing of malposed teeth into correct vertical alignment. This is done with looped archwires or with very light but springy wires.

LIGATURE—In orthodontics a thin steel wire which is used to tie a main arch wire into the bracket which is attached to the tooth. Plastic ligatures and self locking brackets that require no liagtures at all have recently been developed.

LINGUAL—In the direction of the tongue.

LINGUAL ARCH—An orthodontic wire contoured to conform to the tongue side of teeth usually connecting lower cuspids or lower first molars. It may be soldered or hooked to bands and is chiefly used as a holding or retaining device.

LYMPH NODES—Nodules occurring in many places in the body where white lymphatic fluid is aggregated. A chief function of the lymphatic system is to fight the invasion of disease carrying organisms.

MALOCCLUSION—Any of the various malpositions of teeth. (See Angle classification.)

MANDIBLE—The lower jaw.

MAXILLA—The two jaws bones are the Superior and Inferior Maxillae. When used without qualification, maxilla is generally understood to mean the upper jaw.

MESIAL—Toward the front or midline.

METABOLISM—The sum of all the physical and chemical activities by which living things are produced and maintained and also the process in which energy is derived from food and utilized by the organism.

MODELS—Reproductions in plaster of sets of teeth. Sometimes called casts.

MOLAR—A posterior grinding tooth.

MONOBLOC—One of the activator type appliances whose purpose is to change the bite by altering reflex pathways.

MUTATION—A sudden change in a gene causing the appearance of a new characteristic in succeeding generations. Most mutations are harmful.

NEUROSIS—A relatively mild form of mental disease.

NORMAL DISTRIBUTION—A description of the frequency with which things happen in the realm of biology. The normal distribution also characterizes the occurrence of many other "variables" throughout the universe. It follows the normal curve, a symmetrical, bell shaped representation of probability.

NUCLEUS—The vital center of most cells which controls their growth, metabolism, and. through its possession of chromosomes, the transmission of genetic qualities.

OCCLUSAL—Toward the biting edge of a tooth.

Glossary 145

OCCLUSION—In dentistry, the way teeth of one jaw meet the teeth of the other jaw.

OPERANT CONDITIONING—A specialized form of behaviorism, developed by B. F. Skinner, in which animals are successively shaped to behave in a desired way through the use of specified schedules of reinforcement. The reinforcement may be positive in the form of a reward or negative in the form of a painful or noxious stimulus. In operant conditioning reinforcement is applied immediately after the desired response, not before it, as in classical conditioning.

ORTHODONTICS (formerly, orthodontia)—The branch of dentistry concerned with the correction of irregular, spaced, or poorly occluding teeth.

ORTHOPEDICS—The branch of medicine treating disorders of the spine, bones, joints, muscles or other parts of the skeletal system.

OVERBITE—A type of malocclusion in which upper incisor teeth vertically overlap the lower teeth. Because of this overclosure, mandibular incisors may bite near or even into the soft tissue of the palate.

OVERJET—The extent to which the upper incisor teeth protrude in the horizontal plane from the lower incisor teeth.

PALATE—The roof of the mouth consisting of the anterior, hard palate formed by the maxillary and palatine bones and their thin covering of soft tissue and the posterior soft palate which has no bony base. The palate separates the oral from the nasal cavity or, to put it another way, the roof of the mouth *is* the floor of the nose.

PEDODONTICS—The specialty dealing with dental disease in children.

PERIODONTAL LIGAMENT—The periodontal ligament or membrane is the soft connective tissue which surrounds teeth in their bony crypts. Some periodontal fibers connect the cementum of the root with the bone of the jaws. Other fibers join the ligament of one tooth with that of another.

PERIODONTICS—The dental specialty treating diseases of the gums or periodontium.

PLACEBO—A substance with no healing properties administered, as a medicine, for its emotionally soothing effect or as a control in an experiment testing the action of another drug supposed to have a real biological action.

PLAQUE—A gelatinous accumulation of bacteria and food debris that adheres to teeth and is thought to be responsible for diseases of both the gums and the hard parts of teeth. It should be removed daily with a toothbrush and dental floss.

PLEASURE PRINCIPLE—In psychoanalysis an instinctual urge for immediate gratification of desires. Tied to deep, wild, and largely unconscious drives, the PLEASURE PRINCIPLE serves the needs of immature areas of personality as opposed to the REALITY PRINCIPLE which operates in harmony with the mature understanding of the conscious mind.

POSITIONER—A flexible mouthpiece made of rubber or plastic which is constructed on an idealized set of models of the patient's teeth. Worn approximately four hours a day after the close of active orthodontic treatment, the positioner is capable of teasing a patient's improved teeth into an even better alignment.

PROGNATHISM—Protrusion of a jaw.

Glossary

PROGNOSIS—A prediction of the probable course and outcome of a disease or disorder.

PROTRUSION—A prominence or projection as of teeth that incline forward excessively from the mouth.

PUBERTY—The time of life in which a person becomes capable of sexual reproduction of children, as opposed to cloning, which is more efficient but less fun. In common law the magic age is presumed to be 14 for males and 12 for females.

PSYCHOSIS—A serious mental disorder in which the patient shows severe change, disorientation, or disorganization of the personality and is said to be "out of touch with reality."

PULP—The vital center of a tooth, sometimes loosely referred to as the "nerve." In addition to nerve endings, the pulp also contains blood and lymphatic vessels that communicate with their respective vascular and nervous systems in the rest of the body.

RAMUS—A branch. In dental anatomy, the ascending portion of the mandible. The horizontal part of the lower jaw, which houses the teeth, is the body.

REALITY PRINCIPLE—In psychoanalysis, the mature conviction that postponement of immediate gratification can likely lead to delayed but more substantial rewards and avoid painful consequences.

REINFORCEMENT—In operant conditioning a reward or punishment delivered immediately after completion of the desired performance.

REFLEX—An involuntary response to a stimulus resulting from the delivery of a circular message through the nervous system. A nerve ending registers the stimulus and transfers the impulse to the central nervous system which sends back a command to a nerve ending attached to a muscle which, in turn, effects the response, a knee jerk or salivary excretion, for example, as in the case of Pavlov's dogs. This round trip is known as a reflex arc.

REMOVABLE APPLIANCE—An orthodontic device that a patient inserts or removes himself. Some are designed to accomplish basic tooth moving objectives, while the action of others is limited to the maintenance or consolidation of previous achievements.

RETAINER—An orthodontic device programmed to prevent the relapse of straightened teeth toward their earlier erring status. Usually made of acrylic and removable, retainers can also be of the fixed variety and cemented in place.

ROOT—The part of the tooth encased in bone.

ROOT CANAL FILLING—When advanced caries or a sharp blow or some other mishap causes the pulp of a tooth to die, either the tooth itself or the pulp alone must be sacrificed. If the tooth is to be retained, the pulp is removed and in its place a root canal filling is inserted, a service that is performed by the family dentist or a specialist called an endodontist.

SEPARATOR—A spring or twisted wire placed between teeth to force them apart, more or less gently, so that shortly thereafter an orthodontic band can be fitted and or cemented into place without the let or hindrance of a tightly touching next door neighbor tooth.

SERIAL EXTRACTION—The planned, orderly removal of teeth so that each newly arrived tooth will find sufficient space in the oral cavity to feel at home. Usually a permanent

Glossary

tooth will eventually be extracted, at the proper time, in each of the four corners of the mouth.

SPACE MAINTAINER—A device used to prevent adjacent teeth from drifting into the vacuum left when a deciduous tooth is lost prematurely. Space maintainers are usually fixed.

STIMULUS—In medicine, something that excites an animal, or part of an organism, into activity.

STRIPPING—The gentle sanding away of the sides of teeth to make them thinner. This is one way that a moderate crowding can be relieved.

SUCCEDANEOUS TEETH—Something that is succedaneous substitutes for something else. Thus, permanent teeth are succedaneous . . . they replace baby teeth.

SUPERNUMERARY TEETH—The dental formula for man includes 32 permanent teeth. Sometimes they do not all form while occasionally one or more *extra* teeth crop up. Most of these interlopers are poorly formed but some are indistinguishable from the normal complement. These extra teeth are supernumeraries.

SURGICAL ORTHODONTICS—In this new way of correcting malpositioned teeth, whole sections of jaw bone are removed or shifted to new places.

SUTURE—The line of meeting of two bones. Eventually the sutures of the skull harden but in the early years of life the sutures consist of soft tissue, an arrangement which permits orthopedic movement.

TEMPEROMANDIBULAR JOINT—The articulation between the mandible and the temple (temporal) bone.

TONGUE THRUST—A habit, usually associated with swallowing, in which the tongue is vigorously propelled between the parted teeth of the two jaws. It is thought to contribute to a failure of opposing teeth to meet, an open bite.

Tube—The attachment welded to the most distal band in the arch. Into it the arch wire is slipped. The other teeth carry brackets into which the main wire is tied or pinned.

Unconscious—In psychoanalysis, the part of the mind containing material of which the waking mind, the ego, is unaware.

Variable—A quality or substance that may assume different values, that is free to vary. Because it can be counted or weighed a variable is the fundamental unit of statistical research.

REFERENCES AND NOTES

Introduction—

1. Bettelheim, B., *The Informed Heart*, Glencoe, Ill., The Free Press, 1960.

Chapter One—From Ancient Egypt to Health Insurance, A Short History of Orthodontics

1. Fox, J., *The Natural History and Diseases of the Human Teeth*, 2nd Ed., London, E. Cox and Son, 1814.
2. Case, C., "Principles of Retention in Orthodontics," *Dental Items of Interest*, Jan.-Feb, 1921.
3. Hixon, E., and Klein, P., "Simplified Mechanics: A Means of Treatment Based on Available Scientific Information," *Am. J. Orthod.*, 62:113-141, 1972.
4. Dickson, G.C., *Orthodontics in General Dental Practice*, 2nd Ed., Philadelphia, Lea and Febiger, 1964.

Chapter Three—The Emotional Importance of Teeth

1. Drennan, R.E., *The Algonquin Wits*, New York, The Citadel Press, 1968.
2. Greenburg, D., *How to be a Jewish Mother, A Very Lovely Training Manual*, Los Angeles, Price, 1964.
3. Schowalter, J.E., "The child's reaction to his own terminal illness," in, *Loss and Grief, Psychological Management in Medical Practice*, Schoenberg, B., Carr, A.C., Peretz, D., and Kutscher, A., (Eds), New York, Columbia University Press, 1970.
4. Berscheid, E., and Walster, "Beauty and the Beast," *Psychology Today*, 5:42:46, March, 1972.
5. Rosenthal, R., and Jacobson, L. *Pygmalion in the Classroom: Teacher Expectation and Pupil's Intellectual Development*, New York, Holt, Rinehart, and Winston, 1968.
6. Knorr, N. J., Hoopes, J. E., and Edgerton, M. T., "Surgical Approach to Adolescent Disturbances in Self-Image," *Plast. and Reconst. Surg.* 41:3, 1968.
7. Down, L., quoted in Kingsley, N.W., *A Treatise On Oral Deformities*, New York, D. Appleton and Co., 1880.

CHAPTER FOUR—Workers in the Field: Who Treats Malocclusion?

1. Angle, E.H., *Treatment of Malocclusion of the Teeth*, 7th Ed., Philadelphia, S. S. White Dental Manufacturing Co., 1907.

CHAPTER SIX—The Diagnostic Decision 2: To Extract or Not to

1. Senet, A., *Man in Search of His Ancestors*, New York, McGraw-Hill, 1956.
2. Angle, E.H., *Items of Interest*, 1903.
3. Angle, E.H., *Treatment of Malocclusion, op. cit.*
4. Wuerpel, E. H., "Processes of the Mind," *Angle Orthodontist*, 2:51-65, 1932.
5. Angle, E.H., *op. cit.*
6. Wuerpel, *op. cit.*
7. Lash, J., *Eleanor and Franklin, the Story of their Relationship Based on Eleanor Roosevelt's Private Papers*, New York, W.W. Norton, 1971.
8. Macgregor, F.D., "Social and Psychological Implications of Dentofacial Disfigurement," *Angle Orthodontist*, 40:231-233, 1970.
9. Colyer, J.F., *John Hunter and Odontology*, London: Claudius Ash, Sons, & Co., Ltd., 1913.
10. Mandel, I., Fall, 1973, Personal Communication.

    According to Irwin Mandel, a professor at Columbia who has undertaken pioneering studies of the bio-chemistry of the oral environment, the potential risk of stripping lower anterior teeth is not great. The minerals rubbed off by the abrasive are quickly replaced by the saliva in which these teeth are bathed. Remineralization is slower to occur for posterior teeth but this omission can be corrected by the dentist. He has only to give them one or two applications of a topical fluoride treatment to restore their original hardness.
11. Farrel, E., "Dentistry's Past and Future Meet in Egypt," *J.A.D.A.*, 86:553-562, 1973.

    Interesting confirmation of the theory that man's snout is receding while his brain case advances in the process of evolution was obtained in 1965 by a team of anthropologists and orthodontists who used cephalometric radiography to compare the ancient Nubian population of the Nile valley, representatives of which were then still available in the form of mummies, with their present day descendants. After the University of Michigan team assembled its computerized records the necropolis at Abu Simbel disappeared under the waters of Lake Nasser which had been created by the Aswan High Dam project. The data, according to Eileen Farrel's article in the

March, 1973 issue of the *Journal of the American Dental Association,* "supports the hypothesis that man's face is becoming smaller through time at a greater rate than his teeth, with dental crowding as the apparent result."
12. Begg, P.R., "Stone Age Man's Dentition," *Am. J. of Orthodont.,* 40 :298-312, 373-383, 462-475, 517-531, 1954.

CHAPTER EIGHT—Final Diagnostic Adventures: The Doctor's Dilemma.

1. Angle, *op. cit.*
2. Graber, T. M., *Orthodontics, Principles and Practice,* 3rd Ed., Philadelphia, W. B. Saunders, 1972.
3. Hixon, E.H., "Cephalometrics: a Perspective," *Angle Orthodontist,* 42 :200-211, 1972.
4. *Ibid.*

CHAPTER NINE—Dental Data

1. In a letter published in the *New York Times* (March 22, 1973) Ernest Hausman, Professor of Oral Biology at the State University of New York at Buffalo, neatly summed up our current understanding of the process of dental decay. Here is the plot outline as he sees it, "Bacteria aggregated on tooth surfaces (dental plaque) utilizing dietary sugar as an energy source produce acid which dissolves the tooth in localized areas. Obviously sugar is not the only factor, but one of a triad of factors: bacteria, diet and susceptible tooth.
Therefore, the most effective control of dental decay involves trying to influence each component of this triad; mechanical cleansing for plaque control, ffuoride making the tooth less susceptible to acid attack, and dietary restrictions of sugar to reduce the acid production by plaque bacteria." Hausmann urged a reduction in the sugar content of the foods served to America's young people. His recommendations apply with extra force to orthodontic patients.

CHAPTER TEN—The "Right" Age to See the Orthodontist

1. Tweed, C.H., *Clinical Orthodontics,* St. Louis, C. V. Mosby, 1966.

CHAPTER ELEVEN—Molar Mechanics: What All Those Little Gadgets are For and How They Work.

1. Hixon and Klein, *op. cit.*
2. While some harried suburban mothers may feel that once a month visits to the orthodontist recur too frequently, it should be noted that things were once much worse. In his 7th edition (1907), Angle advised "experienced operators" to see their patients once a week and "inexperienced operators" to see them twice a week.

3. Hixon, *op. cit.*
4. Begg, P.R., *Begg Orthodontic Theory and Technique*, Philadelphia, W. B. Saunders, 1965.

CHAPTER TWELVE—But Sometimes Those Gadgets Don't Work at All. How Come?

1. Blos, P., Oct. 2, 1972, Personal communication.
2. Although it may appear that the author is referring to himself, he is actually quoting his cousin, who is in the same line of work. Weiss, Jerome, October, 1973, Personal communication.
3. Campisi, R.S., "A Study of Truthfulness in Male Orthodontic Patients from the Appraisal of Certain Autonomic Responses to Questions Concerning Cooperation," Unpublished master's thesis, Loyola University, 1963.
4. Cavanaugh, Jr., T.P., "A Study of Truthfulness in Female Orthodontic Patients," Unpublished master's thesis, Loyola University, 1963.
5. Weiss, J., "Some Psychological Aspects of Dental Pain," *N.Y. State Dent. Journal*, 38 :32-35, 1972.
6. Kaye, S.R., "Detecting Caries on Film Without Removing Bands," *Dental Survey*, November, 1972, page 38.
7. Gannon, M.F., "Formation and Administration of an Attitude Scale for Orthodontic Patients," Unpublished master's thesis, Loyola University, 1964.
8. Montandon, D., "A quel âge doit-on operer les malformations congenitales de la face?," *Médècine et Hygiene*, 1002 :406-407, March, 1972.
9. Fraiberg, S.H., "Homosexual Conflicts," in Lorand, S. and Schneer, H., *Adolescents—Psychoanalytic Approach to Problems and Therapy*, New York, Harper and Row, 1961.
10. Essig, J., December, 1973, Personal communication.
11. *Ibid.*
12. Campisi, Cavanaugh, and Gannon, *op. cit.*
13. Carr, A.C., and Schoenberg, B., "Object-Loss and Somatic Symptom Information," in Schoenberg, B., Carr, A.C., Peretz, D., and Kutscher, A. (Eds.), *Loss and Grief: Psychological Management in Medical Practice*, New York, Columbia University Press, 1970.
14. Janis, I., and Feshbach, S., "Effects of Fear Arousing Communications, *Journal of Abnormal and Social Psychology*, 48 :78-92, 1953.
15. Crowder, T.H., Jr., *The Dental Student and Social Responsibility: a Review of the Literature*, Chicago, American Association of Dental Schools, 1966.

16. Sherlock, B.J., and Morris, R.T., *Becoming a Dentist*, Springfield, Ill., Charles C. Thomas, 1972.
17. Kelly, J.E., "Twenty-four hours per-day Head Gear, I Like It," Paper delivered at annual meeting of Eastern Association of Strang Tweed Study Groups, New York, December, 1972.
18. Gannon, *op. cit.*
19. Blos, P., *On Adolescence, A Psychoanalytic Interpretation*, Glencoe, Ill., The Free Press, 1962.

CHAPTER THIRTEEN—Now You See Them, Now You Don't: Some Possibilities for the Future.

1. Steffens, L., *The Autobiography of Lincoln Steffens*, New York: Harcourt, Brace & Co., 1931.
2. Newman, G., "Bonding Plastic Orthodontic Attachments to Tooth Enamel," *Journal of the N.J. State Dental Society*, May-June, 1964.
3. Jones, E., *The Life and Work of Sigmund Freud*, Vol. I, New York, Basic Books, 1953.
4. Newman, G., April 1973, Personal communication.
5. *Ibid.*
6. Newman, G., "Bonding Plastic Attachments," *op. cit.*
7. Shaw, B., "The Doctor's Dilemma," in *The Complete Plays of Bernard Shaw*, London, Constable & Co., 1931.
8. Haas, A.J., *"Palatal Expansion, Just the Beginning of Dentofacial Orthopedics,"* Amer. J. Orthodont. 57:219-255, 1970.
9. Graber, T., *Orthodontics, Principles and Practice*, 3rd Ed., Philadelphia, W.B. Saunders, 1972.
10. Sassouni, V., Lecture notes, postgraduate course, University of Pittsburgh, Spring, 1973.
11. Sassouni, V., "Dentofacial Orthopedics: A Critical Review," *Am. J. of Orthod.*, 61:255-269, 1972.
12. Reboul, M., Personal communication, Spring, 1973.

CHAPTER FOURTEEN—The Role of Surgery in Orthodontics, Past, Present, and Future.

1. Dougherty, H.L., "Intraoral Soft Tissue Problems in Orthodontic Practice," *J.A.D.A.*, 82:841-851, 1971.
2. Angle, E.H., *Treatment of Malocclusion of the Teeth and Fractures of the Maxillae*, 6th Ed., Philadelphia, S.S. White Dental Manufacturing Co., 1900.
3. Poulton, D., "The Orthodontic Approach to Class III Malocclusions," *J.A.D.A.*, 82:805-812, 1971.
4. *Ibid.*

5. Russell, B., *Bertrand Russell Speaks His Mind,* New York, The World Publishing Co., 1960.
6. MacIntosh, R.B., "The Surgical Approach to Class II, Division I Malocclusion," *J.A.D.A.,* 82:796-804, 1971.
7. Among those who should be particularly careful to avoid any medication they don't absolutely require are pregnant women. Unborn children are especially susceptible to drugs and it appears that pregnant women everywhere tend to dose themselves heavily. A study in Scotland, according to Jane E. Brody writing in the *New York Times* of March 18, 1973, showed that 82 per cent of women surveyed took medication during their pregnancies, with an "average of four drugs prescribed per woman. Sixty-five per cent of the women took drugs on their own, with an average of 2.2 drugs per woman." And the situation is as bad or worse in this country, Ms. Brody added. Actually no woman in her child-bearing years should use any medication she doesn't have to. Even potential fathers ought to be on the alert since "some drugs may damage the genes carried by sperm cells." And Ms. Brody wasn't just talking about thalidomide. A wide range of chemicals, including the housewife's friend, aspirin, are "suspected of being hazardous and others might be causing subtle damage, such as a decrease in intelligence or behavioral abnormalities that would be very difficult to detect."
8. Mackintosh, *op. cit.*
9. Amato, C., September, 1973, Personal communication.

CHAPTER FIFTEEN—Calculated Risks and Risky Calculations.

1. McGrew, W.C., and Tutin, C.E.G., "Chimpanzee Dentistry," *J.A.D.A.,* 85:1198-1204, 1972.
2. Schmeck, Jr., H.M., "Federal Guideline on Radiation Level is Called Too High," *New York Times,* Nov. 16, 1972.
3. Schmeck, Jr., H.M., "Radiation, How Much is Too Much?" *New York Times,* Nov. 19, 1972.
4. Lupton, D.E., "Psychological Aspects of Temperomandibular Joint Dysfunction," *J.A.D.A.,* 79:131-136, 1969.
5. Perry, H.T., "Relation of Occlusion to Temperomandibular Joint Dysfunction: The Orthodontic Viewpoint," *J.A.D.A.,* 79:37-141, 1969.
6. Loiselle, R.J., "Relation of Occlusion to Temperomandibular Joint Dysfunction: The Prosthodontic Viewpoint," *J.A.D.A.,* 79:145-146, 1969.
7. Laskin, D.M., "Etiology of the Pain-Dysfunction Syndrome," *J.A.D.A.,* 79:147-153, 1969.
8. Bell, W.E., "Clinical Diagnosis of the Pain-Dysfunction Syndrome," *J.A.D.A.,* 79:154-160, 1969.

References and Notes

9. Bell, W.H., "Nonsurgical Management of the Pain-Dysfunction Syndrome," *J.A.D.A.*, 79:161-170, 1969.
10. Marbach, J.J., "Therapy for Mandibular Dysfunction in Adolescents, and Adults," *Am. J. Orthod.*, 62:601-605, 1972.
11. Ricketts, R.M., "The Value of Cephalometrics and Computerized Technology," *Angle Orthodontist*, 42:179-199, 1972.
12. Sassouni, V., "Diagnostic et traitement orthodontique par ordinateur," Report given to the 46th annual session of the Société Française d'Orthopédie Dento-Faciale, Nov. 1973.
13. Ricketts, *op. cit.*
14. Moss, M., "Lecture Notes," Postgraduate Course, Columbia University, Spring, 1972.
14a. Salzmann, J.A., "Reliability of Prediction in Orthodontics" (Editorial), *Am. J. Orthod.* 61:518-519, 1972.
15. Hixon, E.H., "Cephalometrics: a Perspective," *Angle Orthodontist*, 42:200-211, 1972.
16. Moore, A.W., "Cephalometrics as a Diagnostic Tool," *J.A.D.A.*, 82:775-781, 1971.
17. Salzmann, J.A., "Effect of Molecular Genetics and Genetic Engineering on the Practice of Orthodontics," *Am. J. Orthod.*, 61:437-472, 1972.
18. Klein, D., "Les manipulations génétiques-Etat actuel des connaissances et perspectives d'avenir," *Médècine et Hygiene*, Numero 1043: 221-225, Feb. 1973.
19. *Ibid.*
20. *Ibid.*
21. Taylor, G. R., *The Biological Time Bomb*, New York, New American Library, 1968.
22. Salzmann, *op. cit.*
23. Klein, *op. cit.*
24. Pruzansky, S., "Letter to the Editor," *Am. J. Orthod.*, 62:539-542, 1972.
25. Kurtz, P., "Medicine and the State: the First Amendment Violated, an Interview with Thomas Szasz," *The Humanist*, 33, 2: 4-9, March-April, 1973.
26. Throughout medical practice, there has been a growing tendency for doctors to assign duties they formerly looked after themselves to less intensively trained assistants. Dentistry is travelling right along with its sister specialities and orthodontists have been especially active in the movement. There is little doubt that more and more routine orthodontic tasks will be delegated to auxiliary personnel in the future. True, some conservative dentists, many of whom occupy positions of power in the dental establishment, continue to resist. Arrayed against them are most educators, busy practitioners seeking relief

from an overcrowded schedule, and, probably decisively, governmental authority. If it becomes national policy to see that health care becomes available to all, one way to improve delivery of services will be to remove restrictive legislation that prevents well-supervised para-professionals from performing certain treatment tasks.

Such utilization of auxiliaries has obvious advantages for the practitioner: it elevates him from the skilled craftsman category and establishes him comfortably in the role of entrepreneur. His productivity ceases to be limited to what he can accomplish with his own two hands. But there can also be benefits for the patient. After all, an assistant can explain the technique of wearing head gear or elastics just as well as the boss and perhaps more patiently. The same goes for the installation and removal of archwires and much more. Freed from these obligations, an orthodontist has additional time to mull over diagnostic and treatment dilemmas, which is what he has been trained to do. Soon he might even closely approximate Hixon's vision of a liberated diagnostician, not tied down to the "jewelry business." Improved efficiency could thus lead to results superior to previous standards because procedures would be more thoughtfully planned and more thoughtfully executed. Such a development might also provide bored patients cooling their heels in front of a receptionist's desk with something they dearly desire—a reduced waiting time.

Author's Note: In instances where no source is given for remarks, statements, or anecdotes information was obtained through direct conversations with the workers themselves or from letters written by them. Translations of a few quotations taken from articles originally published in French were done by me.

INDEX

Activator, 106-108, 133, 137, 144
Adenoids, 48
Adolescent Personality, The, 87
Adolescents, Psychoanalytic Approach to Problems and Therapy, 91, 154
Adult orthodontics, 81, 82
AMATO, C., 118, 155
Age to begin treatment, 67-72, 81, 82, 95-97, 143
Algonquin Wits, The, 151
American Association of Dental Schools, 94
American Board of Orthodontics, 21
American Dental Association, 4, 20
American Institute of Orthodontists, 20
American Society for the Study of Orthodontics, 20
Anaesthesia, 77, 101, 110, 111, 117
Anchorage, 78, 79, 137
ANGELL, E.C., 103
Angle Classification, 8, 137
ANGLE, E.H., 2, 8, 21, 32-37, 48, 76, 77, 103, 113, 114, 117, 137, 152-155
Anterior component of force, 42
Appearance, facial, 12-17, 33, 51
Arch, 137
Arch wire, 77, 79, 80, 137
Articulation, 56, 137

Bands, 75-77, 79, 80, 100, 138
BARUCH, B., 99, 100
Becoming a Dentist, 94, 155
BEGG, R., 37, 42, 63, 75, 77, 85, 138, 153
Begg technique, 63, 64, 75
Behavior modification, 22, 45, 46, 138
BELL, W.E., 126
BELL, W.H., 126
BENCHLEY, R., 11

BERSCHEID, E., 12, 151
BETTELHEIM, B., viii, 151
BLOS, P., 87, 90, 96, 154, 155
Bite, 2, 3, 6
    closed, 74, 85
    cross, 8, 9, 67, 68, 73, 114-116
    open, 9, 49, 51, 74, 85
    over, 9
Biological Time Bomb, The, 133
Body image, 13-17, 23, 87, 90, 138
Bonding (see Plastic braces)
BOOTH, E., 51
Bracket, 77, 138
Bridge, 40, 82, 138
Bruxism, 47, 48, 139
BUNNY, BUGS, 8, 74, 78
Button, 76, 139

CAMPISI, R.S., 88, 154
Cap, 41, 139, 143
Caries (see Cavities)
CARR, A.C., 93, 154
CASE, C., 2, 103, 151
CAVANAUGH, T.P., JR., 88, 154
Cavities, 2, 61, 64, 65, 121, 122, 139
Cementum, 63, 139
Cephalometric X-Ray, 25, 26, 127, 128, 139
Chromosome, 132, 139
Class I Malocclusion, 8, 71, 137
Class II Malocclusion, 8, 12, 78, 92, 104, 115, 137
Class III Malocclusion, 8, 58, 78, 104, 115, 137, 155
Cleft palate, 9, 56, 140
Cloning, 132, 140
COHN-STOCK, 117
COLYER, J.F., 152
Computers, 128, 129
Condyle, 56, 140
Cooperation, 5, 87-97
Cost of treatment, 2, 3, 29, 86
CRICK, F.H.C., 131, 132
CROWDER, T.H., JR., 94, 154
Cross bite, 67

159

Crowding of teeth, 70, 71
   and decay, 52
   return of, 84
Crown, 60, 61, 64, 122, 140
CROZAT, G., 74, 75

Decalcification, 88, 121, 127, 140, 142
Deglutition, 49, 140
Dentin, 65, 140
Deoxynucleic acid (DNA), 130, 131
Diastema, 60, 112, 141
DICKSON, G.C., 151
Diet, 2, 16, 37, 64, 81, 92, 153
Dishing in, 74, 141
Doctor's Dilemma, The, 103
DOWN, L., 16, 151
Down's syndrome, 17
DRENNAN, R.E., 151
DOUGHERTY, H.L., 112, 155
DYLAN, BOB, viii

EDGERTON, M.T., 14
Edgewise system, 75, 141
EISER, H.M., 96, 97
Elastics, 78, 88, 89, 97, 126, 141, 148
Enamel, 64, 65
Erogenous zone, 16, 141, 142
ESSIG, J., 91-93, 154
Etching (see Decalcification)
Expansion, 22, 36, 71, 74, 142
   rapid, 103-105
Extraction, 2, 21, 23, 31-37, 41, 42, 51, 52, 71, 77
   and facial appearance, 52-54
   and anaesthesia, 110, 111

FARRAR, J., 3, 4
FARREL, E., 152, 153
FESHBACH, S., 94, 154
Finger sucking, 43, 46, 47
FORD, H., 2
Fox, J., 2, 151
FRAIBERG, S., 91, 154
Frenum, 60, 112, 113, 142
FREUD, S., 16, 101, 118, 131
FRIEDMANN, 134

GANNON, M.F., 88, 90, 96, 154, 155
Genetics, 129-134, 142
Gingiva, 7, 61-63, 82, 88, 142
Gingivitis, 62
GRABER, T., 107, 153, 155
GREENBERG, D., 12, 151
Gums (see Gingiva)

HAAS, A.J., 105
Habits, 43-48, 58
HARVOLD, E., 107
HAUSMAN, E., 153
HAWLEY, C., 83
Hawley retainer, 83, 84
Hay rake, 44
Head gear, 79, 81, 88, 91, 95, 97, 142
Heredity, 35, 37, 38, 129-134
HIXON, E., 3, 51, 52, 76, 83, 102, 105, 128, 129, 151, 153, 157
Homo erectus, 31
Homo habilus, 31
Homo sapiens, 39
HOOPES, J.E., 14
How to be a Jewish Mother, 12, 151
HULLIHEN, S.P., 113, 117
HUNTER, J., 35, 152

International Association of Orthodontists, 20
Impaction, 60, 142
Informed Heart, The, viii, 151

Jacket (see Cap)
JACOBSON, L., 13, 151
JANIS, I., 94, 154
Johnson Twin-Arch system, 75
JONES, E., 101

KAYE, S., 89, 154
KELLY, J.E., 154
KINGSLEY, N., 3, 4, 151
KLEIN, D., 133, 157
KLEIN, P., 3, 151, 153
KNORR, N.J., 14, 151
KURTZ, P., 135, 157
KUTSCHER, A., 93, 154

Labio-lingual system, 75
LARDNER, R., 1
LASH, J., 34, 152

Index

LASKIN, D.M., 126
Latency period, 95, 143
Leveling, 77, 78, 143
Lingual arch, 84, 143
Lips, posture of, 25, 26, 28, 36, 37, 40
LOISELLE, R.J., 125
LORAND, S., 91, 154
Loss and Grief: Psychological Management in Medical Practice, 93
Loss of body part, 93, 94
LUPTON, D.E., 125

MACGREGOR, F., 34, 152
MACINTOSH, R.B., 118, 156
MCGREW, W.C., 121, 155
Malocclusion, 3, 4, 6-12, 14, 29, 44, 47, 48
    adult, 81, 82
    relapse of, 84-86, 127, 144
    stability of, 83
    and stigma, 29
Malocclusion of the Teeth, 21, 32
MANDEL, I., 152
Mandible, 31, 56, 79, 144
Man in Search of his Ancestors, 31
MARBACH, J.J., 126
Marx, Groucho, 62, 63
Masturbation, 47
Mauer jaw, 31
Maxilla, 55, 79, 105, 144
Milwaukee brace, 105
Models, plaster, 28, 144
Molecular biology, 129-134
Monobloc (see Activator)
MONTANDON, D., 91, 154
MOORE, A., 128, 129, 157
MORRIS, R.T., 94, 155
Moss, M., 128, 157
Mouth breathing, 48
MULLER, H.J., 130, 131
Musical instruments, 92, 93

Nail biting, 47
NEWMAN, G., 100-103, 155
NEWTON, I., 78, 79, 131
Night brace (see Head gear)
NIRENBERG, M., 133
Normal distribution, 39, 144

OBWEGESER, H., 118
Occlusion, 8, 32
    attritional, 42, 59, 63
    line of, 33, 145
Oedipus complex, 96
On Adolescence, 87
Operant conditioning, 45, 91, 145
Orthodontics in General Practice, 151
Over treatment, 85

Pain, 65, 67, 80, 81, 89, 104
Palate, 55, 56, 103, 104
Parsimony, 115, 116
Patients, cooperation of, 5, 94-97
    number of, 4
Pedodontists, 21, 145
Pencil chewing, 47
PERETZ, D., 93, 154
Periodontal ligament (see Periodontal membrane)
Periodontal membrane, 62, 63, 66, 81, 146
Periodontitis, 62
PERRY, H.T., 125
Phoenician dental patient, 3
Placebo, 126, 146
Plastic braces, 99-102, 112
Plaque, 61, 146
Pleasure principle, 91, 146
Polygraph, 88
Pompeii, 3
Positioner, 84, 85, 146
POULTON, D., 115, 155
Prognathism, 68, 114, 115, 146
Protrusion, 8, 63, 71, 88, 147
    lower, 58, 68, 115, 116
    upper, 58, 68, 69, 85
PRUZANSKY, S., 134, 157
Puberty, 95-97, 147
Psychoanalysis, 4, 16, 44-46, 87, 90, 91, 94-97, 146, 150
Psychosis, 15, 147
Pulp, dental, 65, 147
Pygmalion in the Classroom, 13
Pyorrhea, 63

Reality Principle, 91, 146,
REBOUL, M., 108, 155

REICH, C., vii
Reflex, 50, 147, 148
Resorption, 63, 122, 123
Retainer, 53, 54, 83, 84, 148
Ribonucleic Acid (RNA), 130
RICKETTS, R.M., 128, 129, 157
ROBIN, P., 106
ROBLIN, 134
ROOSEVELT, E., 12, 34, 35, 152
Root canal filling, 65, 66, 148
ROSENTHAL, R., 13, 151
Rubber bands (see Elastics)
RUBENSTEIN, H., 1, 55
RUSSELL, B., 115, 116, 155

SALZMANN, J.A., 129-134, 157
SASSOUNI, V., 107, 108, 128, 155
SCHOENBERG, B., 93, 154
SCHMECK, JR., H.M., 124, 125
SCHNEER, H., 91, 154
SCHOWALTER, J.E., 151
Second opinion, 23
SENET, A., 31, 152
Separators, 75, 148
Serial extraction, 70, 73, 148
SHAW, G.B., 103, 155
SHERLOCK, B.J., 94, 155
Significant others, 13
SKINNER, B.F., 45, 91, 145
SLATER, P., vii
SLOANE, J., 34
Spaces, 67, 70, 74
Space maintainer, 72, 149
Speech therapy, 49-51
Sports, 92
STEFFENS, L., 99, 155
Stigma, 29, 30
Stone age man, 31, 37
Stripping, 37, 42, 54, 71, 85, 149

Supernumeraries, 41, 42, 149
Surgical orthodontics, 113-119, 149
Suture, 56, 104, 149
Swallowing, 49, 50
SZASZ, T., 7, 134, 135, 157

TATUM, E., 133
TAYLOR, G., 133, 157
Teeth, bodily movement of, 74, 75
    deciduous (baby), 2, 56-58
    formation of, 55-62
    number of, 35
    occlusion of, 32
    permanent, 58-60
Temperomandibular joint, 109, 125, 126, 149
Thumb sucking, 2, 43
TOKLAS, A.B., ix
Tongue thrust, 49, 51, 149
Tonsils, 48
Toothbrushing, 64, 122
Treatment, duration of, 5, 81
Tube, 76, 150
TUTIN, C.E.G., 121, 156
TWEED, C., 22, 33, 34, 36, 69, 70, 96, 153

Uniformism, 96
Universal system, 75

WALSTER, 12, 151
WATSON, J.B., 45
WATSON, J.D., 131
WEISS, J., 154
WEISS, JEROME, 87, 88, 154
WUERPEL, E.H., 33, 38, 152

X-rays, 21, 123, 124
    panoramic, 28